THE SCIENCE OF GETTING RIPPED

PROVEN DIET HACKS AND WORKOUT TRICKS TO BURN FAT AND BUILD MUSCLE IN HALF THE TIME

RAZA IMAM

WARNING – Get My <u>Free</u> "Secret" Report

My wife is a registered dietitian and I'm a fitness nut. We regularly send out nutrition tips, fitness hacks, and other health related information. Please sign up for my free newsletter.

I'll also give you a copy of my free report "The ULTIMATE Muscle-Building Dessert"

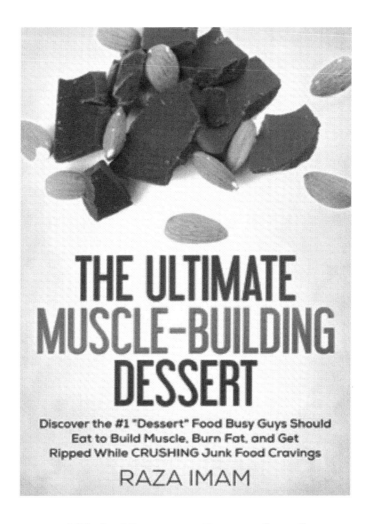

Click Here to Download

https://www.thescienceofgettingripped.com/free-report

http://bit.ly/1UovTv5

Copyright Notice

No part of this report may be reproduced or transmitted in any form whatsoever, electronic, or mechanical, including photocopying, recording, or by any informational storage or retrieval system without expressed written, dated and signed permission from the author. All copyrights are reserved.

Disclaimer and Legal Notices

The information provided in this book is for educational purposes only. I am not a doctor and this is not meant to be taken as medical advice. The information provided in this book is based upon my experiences as well as my interpretations of the current research available. The advice and tips given in this course are meant for healthy adults only. You should consult your physician to insure the tips given in this course are appropriate for your individual circumstances. If you have any health issues or pre-existing conditions, please consult with your physician before implementing any of the information provided in this course. This product is for informational purposes only and the author does not accept any responsibilities for any liabilities or damages, real or perceived, resulting from the use of this information.

Can I Ask You a Quick Favor?

If you like this book, I would greatly appreciate if you could leave an honest review on Amazon.

Reviews are very important to us authors, and it only takes a minute to post.

Also, please check out my newest book:

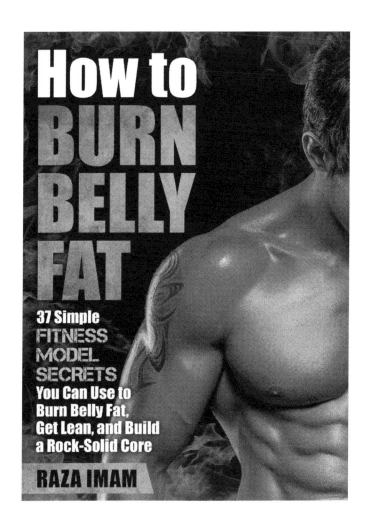

Thank you in advance!

Table of Contents

Acknowledgements 1

Intro 2

Who This Is For 3

My Story 5

What You'll Learn.. 7

What You'll Need: 9

Biggest Mistakes Most Guys Make 10

3 Secrets the Fitness Industry Won't Tell You................... 12

Now Make a Goal 16

The Scientific Formula to Get Ripped 18

What About Calories? 40

Training Principle 1: Training for Strength vs. Training for Muscle Mass 54

Training Principle 2: Fitness is Intensity Dependent, Not Time Dependent 62

Training Principle 3: Compound Full-Body vs. Split Body Part Routines 67

Training Principle 4: The Science of Rest........................ 76

Training Principle 5: The Only REAL Way to Get Abs 84

Training Principle 6: Progressive Overload and Periodization for Progressive Gains 88

Training Principle 7: The "Supreme 7" Movements to Build Muscle, and Lose Fat 94

Training Principle 8: Strength Circuits to Build Muscle and Burn Fat 99

Training Principle 9: High Intensity Interval Training for Fat Loss 109

Training Principle 10: Developing Power 115

Training Principle 11: Cut THEN Bulk? 119

Training Principle 12: The Science of Warming Up 121

Training Principle 13: The Science of the "Deload Week" 125

3 Things to Get Right - Sleep, Water, and Stress Management 129

18 Mindblowing Nutrition Tips for Busy Guys to Get Ripped 164

Free Bonus Report (exclusive for my readers) 182

Acknowledgements

I wanted to thank the following people, without whom I never would have been able to create this book. Their support, advice, insight, and expertise was invaluable in writing.

The following fitness experts have helped me, both directly and indirectly in writing this book. Shawn Lebrun. Rusty Moore. Shin Ohtake. Robert dos Remedios. Craig Ballantyne. Mike Whitfield. Elliott Hulse. Mike Westerdal. Joel Marion. Mike Geary. Mike Ross. Shawna Kaminsky. Ryan Magin. Vince Del Monte. Chad Howse. Nate Green. Steve Kamb. Shawn Hadsall. Eric Wong.

Of course, I wanted to thank my family and friends who supported me, motivated me, and worked out with me while I wrote this. Dave Vela. Majeed Khan. Odeh Neshawait. Chris Smith. Dr. Ali Malick.

Intro

One of my high school teachers once told us the simple keys to success. He was talking about Roger Bannister, the first man to ever run a 4 minute mile. Everyone thought it was impossible and told him he'd never do it. But he didn't care and kept practicing. At the end of the day, accomplishing goals can be broken into 3 simple steps:

1). First you have to do good
2). Then you start feeling good
3). Then you start looking good

I don't care if you're trying to lose weight, be a better parent, learn a new language, or find a new job. You have to take the first step, which means you have to take ACTION. In time, consistent action will lead to confidence and a strong self-image. Then eventually, you, and those around you, will see results.

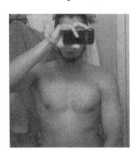 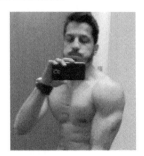

Who This Is For

This is for the average guy who wants to lose fat and build muscle. It's for the busy parent, the entrepreneur, the guy who wants to help others. He needs the physical strength to accomplish his goals, but also the discipline, fortitude, mental toughness, character, and self-respect to handle life's most difficult tasks.

Whether that means turning around a struggling business, volunteering with young kids, or raising a growing family, having a solid physique in addition to the inner strength to blast through life's obstacles and challenges is the key to success.

The ideal reader doesn't want to be a pretty boy fitness model nor a bodybuilder. He reads popular men's health magazines, is interested in technology, and photography, and current events, and sports. He is tech savvy and forward thinking, with aspirations and ambitions for himself and his family. He doesn't want to spend hours a day in the gym. He looks for efficiency and fitness hacks to get him the most results from his workouts.

Here's the thing, most products focus on getting ripped, and this will show you how to do just that. But the way I see it, you don't walk around with your shirt off all day. You DO meet people, solve problems, create plans, help others, encounter obstacles, and live a full life. So why not focus on not only the physical benefits you'll get when you workout, but on the confidence and mental toughness you gain as well? Seems like the best of both worlds to me. .

My Story

Like most 30-something guys with kids, I have a very busy life. Here's my typical day: An hour-long commute to and from work. Helping my 5 year-old with homework. Giving the kids baths. Putting them to bed. Doing dishes. Hanging out with the wife. And going to bed.

I love working out and used to be heavily involved in martial arts. But I just couldn't keep it up with this crazy schedule. I've been wanting to get back in shape for quite a while, but never had the time to go to the gym consistently. Once I hit 30, I was terrified that I would get the dreaded "skinny fat" body type. You know what I'm talking about. Skinny body with a pot belly.

I wanted to get my lean, defined, and muscular body back, but not having enough time was my biggest excuse. Truth is, I mentally gave up. I still wanted to get ripped, but it didn't seem like it was going to ever happen. Because I didn't think I could fit it into my schedule...

I know for a fact that lots of guys can relate.

I did a lot of research and came to realize that guys who want to get ripped need a specific type of workout.

In this report, you'll learn about the workout I followed and the results I was able to achieve.

I hope it helps you in your journey to get lean and ripped. If you follow my advice, I'm sure you will, even if you only have 30 minutes a day.

Sincerely,

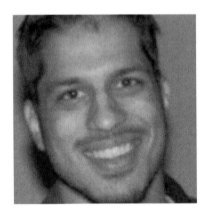

Raza Imam

What You'll Learn

This book is geared towards busy guys who want to get lean and fit as fast as possible. For most guys, especially those with busy lives, and kids, and demanding jobs, their health goes on the back burner. Between helping their kids with homework and attending their sports and other school events, the average American has very little time to dedicate to their health. Add that to a two hour daily commute, and it's easy to see why so many people have a hard time staying in shape. Worst of all is that for guys who do go to the gym after work, it's packed, with most of the exercise equipment occupied. So it's easy to see why people quit their gym memberships just a few months after joining.

This book is written with all of that in mind. I've done a tremendous amount of research and condensed it into simple, actionable information that busy guys like us can use to get into the best shape of their lives. Here's what you'll learn in this book:

1. **How to build a functionally strong body that looks amazing - "show" muscle and "go" muscle**

2. The fastest, most efficient way to get lean and incredibly strong; I'll show you how to gain mass if that's what you want, but the quick workouts will have you in great shape with a minimal time investment
3. Easy to follow workouts that you can do either at home or in the gym
4. How to tweak your workouts to burn fat or build muscle, using the exact same exercises

My goal is to get you noticeable results in the next 15 days so that you're motivated to continue. I know that if you can see and feel the results, you'll look and feel stronger and more confident. Once that happens, others will start to notice and you'll see your life change as a result of your newfound health and fitness.

I once read a quote online that said:

"It takes 4 weeks to see a change in your body. It takes 8 weeks for others to see it. It takes 12 weeks for the world to see it".

What You'll Need:

A membership to the local gym is best. You will be using the power rack (squat rack), barbells, dumbbells, a bench, and pull-up bars. If you can't make it to the gym, then a pull-up bar and dumbbells are going to be all you need. A dip bar is optional but recommended as well.

Biggest Mistakes Most Guys Make

Before we get started, it's important to identify the biggest mistakes most guys make when they're trying to get lean and ripped.

1). Not Having a Plan: Most guys never see any results when they workout because they don't follow a plan. Whether they want to build muscle or lose weight, you have to have a clear, structured workout to help you reach your goals. Most guys just go to the gym and do a bunch of bicep curls, bench presses, and calf raises. They aren't following a plan and that's exactly why they get no results.

2). Doing isolated exercises: Isolated exercises like bicep curls and calf raises don't stimulate enough muscle fibers to build lean muscle or use enough energy to burn lots of calories. It's much better to do full-body, compound exercises with lots of intensity.

3). Using exercise machines: Exercise machines force you into awkward movements. Machines alter how your body naturally moves. This severely limits your ability to activate all of your muscles fibers — so you burn *less* fat and get *less* muscle definition. Free weights are much better because they stimulate hundreds of stabilizer muscles when used properly.

4). Long bouts of "low and slow" cardio: Cardio is important. But there's a right way to do it and a wrong way to do it. When you combine cardio with strength training, you get great results.

5). Doing crunches and setups for a 6-pack: You need to work your core, but remember, abs are made in the kitchen, not in the gym. Proper diet will help you slim down and core exercises will make your abs sharp and defined.

3 Secrets the Fitness Industry Won't Tell You

Before we get started, I wanted to reveal 3 dirty secrets the fitness world keeps under wraps. Understanding these will help you go a long way towards building the body you want.

Secret #1 - Everything Works

If you ask a bodybuilder what the best type of workout is, they might tell you that split-part, bodybuilding workouts with high reps and medium to heavy weights is best. If you ask a strength trainer what the best type of workout is, they might tell you lifting heavy weights 1-5 times is the *only* way to build real strength. If you ask someone who focuses on interval training, they'll tell you that doing multiple exercises that workout your full body with rest is the best way to get lean and muscular.

The truth is that they're all right. If you want to get big and muscular and are comfortable with eating lots of calories, bodybuilding is the way to go. If you care about strength and not about getting big, then focus on strength training. If you want to increase muscular endurance, get better muscular definition, and burn fat, then circuit weight training is perfect for you.

You're a unique person with unique goals. Don't let anyone convince you that one particular way of training is better than the other because they all work. Truth is, all workouts are pretty much the same... more on that below.

Secret #2 - Nothing Works Forever
Here's another dirty truth: most of the fitness industry caters to "newbies". No matter what workout program you follow, if you're overweight, you'll start dropping pounds. If you're skinny and start lifting weights for the first time, you'll notice an increase in strength and will see your physique change. These "newbie" gains major milestones and incredibly motivating.

But the human body is amazing at adapting, so as you progress with your workouts, your body will grow less muscle and will shed less fat unless you change your routine by adding more weights, working out with more intensity, being stricter with your diet, etc.

So make sure you're progressively challenging your body by varying your workout to keep seeing improvement. .

Secret #3 - Most Workouts Are the Same

As you'll learn in the coming chapters, most workouts use the same exercises, or variations of them. These exercises include the bench press, push up, deadlift, row, squat, overhead press, pull up, and dip.

The only real difference between people who want to build muscle and people who want to lose weight is the weight, number of repetitions, rest between sets, and what they eat.

The key is to choose what goal you want to focus on and follow a program that is conducive to that. The more complex your workout is, the less likely you are to do it. So focus on simplicity and efficiency so you can follow your workout consistently.

And remember, since most workouts are the same (except for the 4 factors mentioned above), it's better to work a mediocre plan really well, than to barely work a "perfect" one. My main training principles revolve around 3 main themes:

- Simplicity
- Efficiency
- Intensity

I read on the ScrawnytoBrawny.com blog:

> *"Give me a one-page bullet-list of exactly what I should do. That's worth more to me than a stack of books that I have to dig through to get to the good stuff. I may give you 50 bucks for the books. But I'll pay you $5,000 for the one page."*

That's a quote from Alwyn Cosgrove, a world-famous strength coach and entrepreneur.

Now Make a Goal

In his classic self-help book, "Psycho-Cybernetics", Dr. Maxwell Maltz proved that humans are similar to heat-seeking missiles. Heat-seeking missiles lock onto a target, but what most people don't know is that since most targets are moving, they have to constantly calculate, and recalculate their position until they finally hit their target. In essence, they are always off course, but keep going until they finally "fail" their way to their target.

His assertion was that if you set a goal, focus on it intensely and take action, your mind will literally guide you to achieving that goal. He recommended visualizing the goal, as if it had already been accomplished, and **focusing on the feeling** you would have once you achieve your goal. The combination of a clearly defined goal and strong emotions will help your subconscious mind find a way to achieve it. The example he gave was of an infant reaching for something on a table. At first his hand-eye coordination would be weak. But as he keeps trying, his accuracy improves, until he literally gropes his way to what he wants.

Goal setting is the foundation of any achievement. So take the time to really think about what you want to accomplish with this workout in the next 90 days. *Think about why these are important to you. Think about how you will feel once you accomplish them.*

Make them specific, have a timeframe, and read them every day with conviction, belief that you'll achieve them, and intense desire. This is NOT "new age" wishy-washy stuff. If your goal is realistic, and you have the right motivation, you can achieve anything.

In the next 90 days I would like to:

_____
_____
_____

I will achieve it by:

_____
_____
_____
_____

This is important to me because:

_____
_____
_____

The Scientific Formula to Get Ripped

The most important thing to remember about burning fat and building muscle is that it is scientific. The human body is incredible at storing fat and building muscle when the conditions are right. This book will show you all of the factors and variables involved in "getting ripped".

But before we begin, I want to make one thing very clear: there is no hidden gem that will automatically force your body to burn fat and build muscle. I've consulted with multiple medical doctors and they all agree. There's no "secret" to it. It's just common sense and hard work. And like I mentioned earlier, everything works, and nothing works forever.

I've done a lot of research on this topic, and have presented the simple, scientific steps to burn fat and build muscle. The thing for the average guy like you and me to remember is that there are countless studies on weight loss and muscle gain. If you were to read every single one of them, you'd become overwhelmed and confused. Because many times, scientific research contradicts each other. You might find one study proving why it's good to do cardio for fat loss in a fasted state, while another report will claim the exact opposite. I've done the research and boiled it down to a few basic principles that you can apply to get the best results possible.

So getting ripped is about 2 basic things:

1. **Losing Body Fat**: You need to be between 6% to 12% to actually see your 6 pack
2. **Building/Maintaining Muscle Mass**: Getting ripped is NOT about losing weight, it's about losing fat while still keeping your muscle.

The rest of this chapter will show you how to do these two things so you can build the ripped, powerful body you want.

The Problem with Getting Ripped

before we can discuss getting ripped, you have to assess yourself and your personal situation. So, if you're overweight, with body fat percentage over 20%, you're going to want to focus on burning fat while maintaining your lean muscle. Otherwise, no matter how much muscle you gain, you'll still look overweight, and you'll never get the ripped look you want. If you're underweight and want to gain muscle, you want to maintain your body fat percentage and turn the calories you consume into lean muscle. Each requires two different approaches:

Losing Weight is Easy: Simply consume less calories than you burn. So if your body burns 2000 calories a day, just eat 1800 calories per day and you'll drop 1-2 pounds per week. But you'll likely be losing water and muscle weight, not just fat. So losing weight is easy, but we care about losing fat so your body looks lean and ripped, not losing muscle and water.

Gaining Muscle is Easy: Simple consume more calories than you burn while lifting heavy weights (lifting weights is key). So if your body needs 2500 calories per day when lifting weights, you should consume 2700 calories.

Getting Ripped is Tricky: Getting ripped is tricky because you want to burn fat (which requires you to lower your calories) and build muscle (which requires you to increase your calories), not just "lose weight". So there seems to be a contradiction here because you can't eat more calories and less calories at the same time. It requires understanding how basal metabolic rate, macronutrient breakdown, hormones, cardio, and weight training relate to each other. Luckily, I'll help break that info down as simply as possible. Once you get this, you'll be better than most people who work out in your local gym, allowing you to get awesome results, really fast.

How to Hack Your Metabolism, Macronutrients, Hormones, Cardio, and Weight Training to Get Ripped

Your body is comprised of bone, muscle, organs, blood, and fat. When getting ripped, you need to focus on losing fat, not muscle. Otherwise, you'll end up working out a lot, but looking thin and sickly. Compare Olympic sprinters to marathon runners. Sprinters are lean, muscular, and incredibly athletic. Marathoners on the other hand, have no noticeable muscle mass to show for their hours and hours of training. Of course, they are elite level athletes that have put in tremendous amounts of work to excel at their sport, but they don't have the "ripped" physique most guys want. So suffice it to say, if you want to burn fat, you should train appropriately.

Getting ripped is a balance of a few key factors:

- **Weight Training**: You will not build (or maintain) lean muscle if you don't lift weights
- **Cardio**: You will not burn calories if you don't do high intensity cardio
- **Nutrition**: Understanding the macronutrient breakdown you need to burn fat and build muscle
- **Hormones**: You can literally hack your body's hormonal response once you understand how to combine your nutrition with your weight training and cardio

The next few sections will break down they key scientific concepts you need to. understand in order to engineer your body to burn fat and build muscle.

We'll go over each of these factors

Nutrition

Your body uses 3 main macro nutrients. They are carbs, fat, and protein. In these, you'll have all of your micronutrients like the vitamins and minerals we're all familiar with. Now each macronutrient has its own calorie breakdown. Understanding this will allow you to eat lots of (the right) food without getting fat.

1 gram of protein = 4 calories
1 gram of carbohydrate= 4 calories
1 gram of fat= 9 calories

Understanding how much of each macronutrient you need will help your body get lean and ripped - fast. So let's discuss each one:

Carbohydrates:

Carbohydrates are probably the most popular macronutrients of all. There's tons of hype about carbs and how they make you fat. Hopefully we'll dispel some myths and come to a rational understanding of the role of carbs. There are different types of carbs; complex carbs (potatoes, bread, pasta, etc.) which take your body longer to break down. Then there are simple carbs (table sugar, honey, desserts, etc.) which your body breaks down relatively quickly. Lastly there are fibrous carbs (like vegetables) which your body breaks down slower as well.

At the end of the day, your body turns carbohydrates into a sugar called glucose. When that sugar hits your intestines, it goes to your liver. When your body detects sugar, the pancreas secretes a hormone called insulin. Insulin is critical because it gets sugar out of your bloodstream and into your muscles or your fat stores (depending on the need). This is good because high blood sugar levels is really dangerous. As you'll learn in the section on hormones, you want to control your insulin and how much sugar comes into your system. Otherwise your body will become insensitive to insulin, making it harder to get the sugar out of your blood, this is what happens with Type II Diabetes.

So once your body detects the sugar in your bloodstream, the insulin helps it move into the cells so it can be used for energy. The sugar that is not immediately used is converted to glycogen, which is stored in your muscles for future use. UNDERSTANDING THIS IS CRITICAL TO BURNING FAT AND BUILDING MUSCLE. Your muscles have glycogen stores, so any glucose that isn't use will go into your muscles, but your muscles can only store about 200 grams of glycogen. Your liver stores glycogen too. Anything more than that gets turned into fat. Suffice it to say, insulin is important for metabolizing the sugar in your blood so it goes to your muscles, because if your muscles can't absorb the .glycogen, the body will turn it into fat. Just imagine your fat cells as balloons that fill up and deflate. You can't get rid of fat cells, but you can make sure they don't fill up by keeping your blood sugar low, so it doesn't get converted to fat and fill up your "fat balloon".

So you can eat lots of fibrous carbs like vegetables because they're packed with vitamins and minerals that promote overall health. And they're low calorie, so you can eat tons of vegetables, stay full, and not turn it into fat. I'll discuss how and when to eat complex carbs (whole wheat bread, sweet potatoes, etc.) in just a bit.

The trick is to eat the right type of carbs in the right amounts. So for example, eating lots of complex and fibrous carbs is really good because your body breaks them down slower. So if you eat a fibrous carbohydrate like broccoli, your body will slowly break it down into glucose, causing your pancreas to secrete low levels of insulin to slowly absorb that over time. Whereas if you eat a huge cupcake, your body will turn that into glucose, and because your bloodstream is flooded with sugar, your pancreas will create lots of insulin to absorb that. But since there's so much excess, your body will quickly squirrel it into fat. So you need to eat complex and fibrous carbs so your body slowly turns them into glucose, reducing the chance that it's quickly converted to fat.

Protein:
Your body needs protein to grow. That means growing muscle, finger nails, hair, and even skin. That's why burn victims have such a high protein consumption, regenerating skin is incredibly protein intensive. Also, after water, protein is the most abundant substance found in the human body. Suffice it to say, it is critical for almost every function in your body like growth, and muscle and tissue repair. So having high levels of protein consumption is definitely very healthy and natural.

For our purposes of getting ripped, you'll be lifting heavy weights. This places a tremendous burden on your body, requiring lots of protein. If you don't supply your body with enough protein, your body will start to break it down your muscles into glucose and use that for fuel. This means your body is "catabolic" and breaking itself down. You don't want that because you'll lose muscle mass.

Eating proper amounts of protein is helpful for building muscle, but it's also awesome because 1 gram of protein has only 4 calories compared to fat which has 9 calories. Also, it takes more energy to break down protein. After eating protein, your metabolism increases by about 30%. That means if you eat 100 calories of protein, 30 calories get burned just by digesting and using the protein. Compare that to carbs which use about 10% and fat which burns about 5%. So literally eating protein can help you lose fat.

Some scientists suggest eating one gram of protein per kilogram of your bodyweight, while others say you want to consume 1 gram of protein per pound of bodyweight. If you're lifting weights, you want to cosume about 1 gram per pound of bodyweight per day. So if you weight 175lbs, you want to consume 175 grams of protein to build and maintain lean muscle. This allows a steady stream of amino acids to your muscles so they don't go catabolic and start breaking down your muscle and converting it to glucose.

Fats:

Fat is an often vilified macronutrient, and has taken a lot of heat over the past few decades. As a result, there has been a glut of "low fat" and "fat free" products on the market. Sadly, this has caused more problems than it has solved because to make the products taste good in the absence of fat, the food companies load it up with sugar. And we already discussed that excess sugar in your blood gets converted to fat anyways, so "low fat" and "fat free" means nothing if your body converts the sugar and carbs to fat anyway.

Fats are necessary for the body and critical to many functions, including satiety. So if you strip fat from your diet, you'll constantly feel hungry. When your body detects fat from your diet, it releases a hormone called cholecystokinin (CKK) which tells your "Brain Famine Center" that you're full. If you don't eat any fat, your body will put you in starvation mode and you'll never feel hungry. Also, eating good fats will slow the entrance of carbs into your bloodstream.

Fat is pretty calorie heavy because 1 gram of fat has 9 calories, as opposed to 1 gram of protein which contains 4 calories. So a little goes a long way. The key is to eat healthy fats in the form of peanut butter, almond butter, almonds, olive oil, eggs, and various nuts like walnuts and almonds.

So as far as nutrition is concerned, you want to consume about 40% carbs, 30% protein, and 30% fat to burn fat and build muscle. I'll explain when to eat it so you can actually burn fat and build muscle below.

Weight Training

Weight training is important because it places a demand on your body to rebuild itself. When you lift weights, you're damaging your muscles, requiring more protein to rebuild the muscles to be stronger. You need to lift weights if you want to get ripped because this allows you to have the strong, athletic body of a sprinter, rather than the thin body of a marathon runner.

So lifting weights, along with properly timed protein consumption will fuel your body with the proper amino acids so that your muscles and repair and rebuild themselves. If you don't lift weights and eat enough protein, your body will start breaking down your muscle and your weight loss will consist of lost muscle and water, rather than lost fat.

Cardio

Cardio is another key factor to getting ripped. That's because cardio does a great job of burning body fat. The key to getting the most out of cardio is to train with intensity. As you'll see in a future chapter about high intensity interval training, cardio done at high intensity and brief rest periods is the best for burning fat. So having a moderately high heart rate for 45 minutes isn't all that helpful for burning fat because you're not training hard enough. But doing a short 60 second burst of cardio at a 9/10 intensity level followed by a rest period will cause your heart rate to go up really fast. This will force your body to use both your aerobic energy systems (the one that requires oxygen) and anaerobic energy system (doesn't require oxygen).

If you recall, I mentioned that your muscles can store up to 200 grams of carbs in the form of glycogen. Doing high intensity cardio, your body will use up those glycogen stores. Since glycogen is the unused sugar stored in your muscles, depleting them will force your body to burn fat for energy, as long as you consume enough protein. I'll share a really simple tip on how to do that in a bit.

So because interval training works your aerobic and anaerobic systems, your anaerobic system will uses energy stored your muscles (glycogen aka carbs) for these short, but intense bursts of activity. Your anaerobic metabolism works without oxygen, and the by-product of that work is lactic acid. As lactic acid builds in your body, it creates a state of "oxygen debt" in your body. During recovery periods, your heart and lungs work together to "pay back" this oxygen debt, helping to break down the lactic acid. In this way, your aerobic system uses oxygen to convert carbohydrates to energy. Over time, this is how your body becomes more efficient at delivering oxygen to your muscles, as well as becoming more efficient at compensating for the "oxygen debt" by using oxygen to turn carbohydrates into energy. So interval training cardio (aka sprinting) gets you lean and in shape fast by improving oxygen utilization at the muscular level.

Hormones

Insulin:
Insulin is the hormone that is created when sugar is present in your blood. If your glycogen stores in your muscles are empty (after cardio or weight training), this is good because your body will send the sugar in your blood (glucose) to your glycogen stores in your muscles.

Growth Hormone:
This is the hormone that breaks down fat and builds muscle. As you'll learn in a later chapter, you trigger growth hormone by lifting weights, doing intense cardio, and sleeping.

T3/Thyroid:
Your thyroid is the master gland of your metabolism. If this drops, your body fights the fat loss process.

Leptin:
Leptin is a hormone that basically controls fat loss. It tells your brain and your body to either store fat or burn fat. Some people have called it your hunger hormone. When you eat, your body releases leptin to let you know you're full. Like T3, if this drops, it retards the fat loss process because your body goes into starvation mode and tries to hold on to fat.

The Problem with Going Too Low on Carbs

The problem with going too low on carbs is that you put your body in starvation mode and throw your T3 and leptin levels off. Lots of people tout the "low carb" approach, but the problem is that when your carbs go too low, you lose lots of water. That's because every gram of carbohydrate holds up to 3 grams of water. So if you drop your carbs over a long period of time, you drop your water levels. So you basically lose a lot of water weight. Now you will lose weight, but at the same time, you your body holds on to fat. So you think you're losing weight for the first 2 weeks (mostly water weight), but then your weight loss stops. And instead you start gaining fat because your leptin and T3 is off. Plus, going too low on carbs for too long messes with your brain function which then forces your body to go into a ketogenic state (which we won't discuss here).

5-7 grams of carbs per pound of body weight is recommended by top nutrition experts for people who are lifting heavy weights. For a 165 pound man, that's about 350 grams of carbs per day. That is WAY too much for a sedentary person, but for someone looking to build muscle and get strong, that's an appropriate amount of carbs so your muscle glycogen reserves are full. Otherwise, your body will start burning your muscle tissue to provide the glucose needed for muscular contractions that they aren't getting from glycogen reserves. This will make you look skinny-fat, and you'll never build the lean, ripped body you want.

When glucose is too low, your body will use fat and protein for energy. So your body will cannibalize itself and burn muscle protein just to keep up. So yes, you can manipulate your carb intake for a little while, but you will lose muscle weight and water weight. This will cause you to still look skinny-fat and you'll never get lean and ripped.

So you can and still should eat carbs to keep your hormones in check. I'll explain exactly how to do that in the next section.

Putting It All Together to Hack Your Body into Getting Ripped

Now here's the secret to combining cardio, weight training, hormones, and nutrition to get the body you want.... TIMING. That's it. Simply timing these 4 variables will help you get lean and ripped easily.

Here's how this works:

	Exercise	**Food**
Mon	Lift Weights	More carbs, less fat
Tue	High Intensity Cardio	Less carbs, more fat
Wed	Lift Weights	More carbs, less fat
Thurs	High Intensity Cardio	Less carbs, more fat
Fri	Lift Weights	More carbs, less fat
Sat	High Intensity Cardio	Less carbs
Sun	Rest	

This is called carb cycling. So you don't completely remove carbs from your diet. You simply space them out so your body uses them appropriately.

High Carb Days:
You will eat about 250-350 grams of carbs on these days. That way you fill your muscles with glycogen, so that they can fuel your muscle growth. Of course, you want to be eating about 1 gram of protein per pound of bodyweight, but eating enough carbs will prevent your body from cannibalizing itself and breaking down muscle tissue. Remember, you want to feed the muscle and burn the glucose for energy. You can eat complex carbs like bread, pasta, potatoes, whole grains, oatmeal, etc. on these days. So on the days you lift weights, eat lots of starchy carbs with lots of protein, vegetables, and healthy fats.

Low Carb Days:
On these days you'll eat about 50-100 grams of carbs. You want them to mostly be from fruits and vegetables. That's because every gram of fiber offsets one gram of carbs. So an apple has 19 grams of carbs and 3 grams of fiber, meaning it has a net of 16 grams of carbs. This also helps with fat loss by tricking your body into burning fat for fuel instead of carbs. It also improves your body's response to insulin, increasing your muscle building response. On your cardio days, don't eat starchy carbs, but you can continue to eat protein, vegetables, and healthy fats. That's it, just remove the starchy carbs like rice, oatmeal, bread, pasta, etc. and eat more

vegetables, healthy fats like nuts and avocados, and proteins like meat and fish. This way you burn your body's fat stores and still stay full. Remember, 1 gram of protein has only 4 calories, and about 30% of your calories from protein are burned just to metabolize the protein, so by eating adequate protein, you can eat more and still burn fat!

Timing of Your Carbs:

When you lift heavy weights, you reduce your blood sugar levels. Your glycogen stores a depleted from the heavy workout and are desperately looking to be refueled. This is when you can eat a high amount of simple carbs. That way your body can break the carbs down very quickly. Eating simple carbs right after a heavy weight lifting workout gives your body an insulin spike. This insulin puts your body in a state of muscle building. If you don't get the right amount of nutrients, your body will go into a catabolic state and start breaking down muscle.

The best way to do this is to drink a protein shake 30 minutes after lifting weights. The protein shake should have high amounts of protein and simple carbohydrates like fig newton's, a banana, etc. But protein powder in a fruit smoothie is the most common (and tasty) way to do this. That way it triggers a quick insulin response, which will shuttle the nutrients into your muscles.

Two hours after your weight training workout you can resume eating meals with lots of protein (chicken, fish, beef, etc.) with lots of complex and fibrous carbs like vegetables, potatoes, pasta, bread, etc.

I learned this simple carb strategy from Nate Green over at ScrawnytoBrawny.com He calls it "Simple Carb Cycling". So rather than removing carbs from your diet altogether and wreaking havoc on your hormones (leading to fat gain), you just space out your carbs between weight lifting and cardio days. Manipulating your carbohydrate intake in this manner allows your body to use fat stores for energy production. On the cardio days, you'll restrict complex carbs (bread, pasta, etc.), so your body will burn fat and save muscle as long as you're eating adequate amounts of protein. On the weight lifting days, you'll eat lots of carbs (simple carbs with protein right after your workout and complex carbs like vegetables and bread and pasta in your other meals). Again, complex carbohydrates are good because they break down slower, and don't flood your blood with sugar. But you do want simple carbs right after your workout because in this case you DO want a quick release of sugar in your blood, so it turns to glucose and then goes to your muscles in the form of glycogen.

So when you take in carbs after your workout, your carbs will be used as energy to restore glycogen and build muscle. You want to take in carbs with protein so those carbs aren't converted to fat and so the nutrients from the protein go into the muscle cells to aid growth.

What About Calories?

In general, to lose weight, you need to be at a caloric deficit. The problem is that if you go too low on the calories you'll lose muscle mass. Here's an easy way to calculate the number of calories you need. First determine your body fat percentage. You can do this with an electronic scale. There are other more accurate ways to do this which you can search on the internet, but for simplicity's sake, just use an electronic scale.

Once you have your body fat percentage, you'll need to multiply that by your total bodyweight. For example, if you weight 200 lbs. and have 25% body fat, then 200 x .25 = 25lbs of body fat, meaning you have a lean body mass of 175 lbs. You'll convert your lean body mass to kilograms by dividing by 2.2. So 175/2.2 = 79.55 kilograms of lean body mass. Then you plug that into this formula to determine your basal metabolic rate (BMR):

BMR = 370 + (21.6 x your Lean Body Mass in kilograms)

Then, multiply your Basal Metabolic Rate by an activity factor to calculate your daily energy expenditure:

Activity factor

Light activity = BMR x 1.375 (light exercise/sports 1-3 days/week)

Moderate activity = BMR x 1.55 (moderate exercise/sports 3-5 days/week)

Heavy activity = BMR x 1.725 (heavy exercise/sports 6-7 days/week)

Here are my favorite two app's to calculate calories, macros, and activity levels:

www.1percentedge.com/ifcalc

www.iifym.com/iifym-calculator

If you follow the workouts in this book, you'll be doing strength training 3 times per week and high intensity cardio intervals 3 times per week, so it's safe to assume that you'll be "moderately active". If you don't like cardio (like me) you should still do it because it has a ton of benefits (you'll see in a future chapter). But you absolutely don't do cardio, then use the "light activity" factor. .

Lastly, you'll set your caloric deficit to about 20% below your daily caloric needs. So based on the above calculations:

BMR = 370 + (21.6 x 79.55kg) = 2088

2088 x 1.55 (moderate activity factor) = 3236 daily calories needed

3226 daily calories x .20 = 647

3236 – 647 (20% calorie reduction) = 2589 daily calories needed to lose fat

Of course, you want to keep your macronutrient breakdown as follows to continue to burn fat and build muscle. Remember, be sure to time your carb and protein intake after your intense weight lifting workouts to maintain lean muscle.

- 30% protein
- 30% fat
- 40% carbs

Remember to consume a quick digesting carb source with protein (like a fruit shake) after your weight lifting session on your high carb days.

Key Takeaways

- Eat a healthy diet of 40% carbs, 30% protein, and 30% fats

- On weight lifting days you can eat lots of healthy complex carbs (bread, pasta, etc.) and you should ALWAYS eat lots of fibrous carbs (vegetables). But right after your workout, drink a smoothie with lots of simple carbs (fruit smoothie) mixed with protein powder. Science has proven that drinking a blended high protein and high carb shake after a weight lifting workout will increase growth hormone and insulin dramatically. In this case, insulin is good because it will cause the glycogen and nutrients to go into your muscles.

- On cardio days, you want to limit the amount of carbs you eat to just fibrous carbs like vegetables. That's because carbs get turned into glucose, which triggers insulin production. Insulin shuttles glucose out of your blood and into your muscles. If your muscles are already full of glycogen (glucose), then it will get turned into fat. So insulin is the ultimate anabolic storage hormone, but you want it to be present after working out, otherwise your body won't burn fat. Because insulin is a growth/storage hormone, your body won't effectively burn fat in the presence of insulin. So take out the carbs so you don't produce lots of insulin on these days. Also, if you do cardio in a slightly fasted state, your glycogen reserves will be empty, forcing your body to burn fat for energy. The fear is that you may burn up muscle. The trick around that is to consume 5-10 grams of essential amino acids (or protein) before your cardio so you have enough protein, so your body doesn't tap into the muscle tissue and burns fat instead.

At the end of the day, there are tons of studies and research out there. You want to just stick with a simple plan that you can fit into your busy life. This "carb cycling" approach where you eat high carbs on weight lifting days and low carbs on cardio days is just the trick most busy guys need to get lean and ripped fast.

.

What About Supplements?

At some point in most guys training regimen, they ask the question *"what supplements should I take?"* I'm going to try to answer that question here as simply as I can. After all, the supplement industry is a multi-million (if not multi-billion) dollar industry. You could literally write an entire book about nutritional supplements:

- weight loss supplements
- muscle building supplements
- digestive health supplements
- skin health supplements
- sexual health supplements
- sleep supplements
- vitamin and mineral supplements
- and the list goes on...

You get the picture, there is *no* shortage of supplements that you can buy for a wide variety of ailments and conditions. Peeople get caught into the flawed thinking that they can take pills to magically make their problems disappear, but that is not the case. At the end of the day, nothing replaces healthy eating, proper sleep, adequate water, and stress management. Nothing. You can take all the supplements in the world, but if you aren't drinking enough water, staying up all night, and eating fast food, your body will not get lean and ripped.

With that said, the intelligent and informed use of supplements is helpful to *supplementing* your health. For example, vitamin E is known to reduce prostate and colon cancer. Calcium and vitamin D reduces the risk of osteoporosis in elderly women. Zinc lozenges treat upper respiratory pharyngitis better than most prescriptions. For athletes and fitness minded people, supplements like branch chained amino acids improve recovery, whey protein isolate helps with post-workout recovery, glutamine can help with "overtraining syndrome", and things like chondroitin can help relieve aching joints.

With that said, there are a few supplements that busy guys who want to get ripped could benefit from. I'm not going to go into detail on every single type of supplement there is, but I will breakdown some of the most common ones that busy guys who want to get lean and ripped should be aware of:

Branch Chained Amino Acids

What They Are:
BCAA's are the three most critical amino acids; leucine, isoleucine, and valine. Amino acids are the building blocks of protein. They're called "branch chained" because each one has a fork-shaped outgrowth that looks like a branch. They're unique to all other amino acids because when your body ingests amino acids or whole protein, they get absorbed by the intestines and sent to the liver. Your liver then decides to send break them down and send them to the rest of your body for energy, or it could decide to send them to repair and build muscle tissue. BCAA's though are unique because they tend to be spared by the liver and get direct access to muscle fibers. The muscle fibers themselves make the determination of whether to use them to fuel the fibers for exercise, or to use them to rebuild and repair.

Why They're Helpful:
- They're an alternative energy source for almost all tissue in your body, including muscle
- They promote protein synthesis, which leads to muscle growth by activating a complex called mTOR which speeds up muscle growth. This also prevents the breakdown of muscle tissue when you work out, which is key to getting ripped
- Studies have shown that taking 10 grams of BCAA's before working out caused the body to produce growth hormone 95% higher than those who didn't take them, allowing their bodies to burn more fat and build more muscle

Caffeine
What It Is:
Yes, I'm talking about caffeine that is found in coffee and most teas. You already know what I'm talking about so let's talk about why it's good for you

Why It's Helpful:
- It's a mild stimulant and diuretic causing you to be more alert and urinate more (respectively)
  - It is thermogenic, meaning that caffeine has the ability to rev up your cells, causing them to produce more heat at the cellular level. This means that your fat stores are mobilized, releasing free fatty acids into your bloodstream to be used as energy by your other cells

Creatine
What It Is:

I'm from Chicago, and back when I was in high school, there was a home run competition between Sammy Sosa of the Chicago Cubs and Mark McGuire of the St. Louis Cardinals. Mark McGuire ended up getting more home runs that year (and the Cubs of course never making it to the World Series), there was a lot of controversy surrounding Mark McGuire's use of creatine. As controversial as it was back then, I hear about creatine all the time now.

Creatine is a combination of 3 amino acids: arginine, glycine, and methionine that is naturally found in foods like meat and fish. It can naturally be created by the body by assembling these amino acids, they are used by other proteins, so the body doesn't naturally try to create creatine because these amino acids are used for other functions by your body.

Why It's Helpful:
- Creatine acts as a "shuttle" molecule for phosphorus during muscle contraction by efficiently generating ATP (ATP is the "currency" of energy in the human body)
- When you take oral creatine supplements, it's taken into the muscle cells where it binds with a phosphorus molecule to create creatine phosphate. The more phosphorus the creatine has, the more energy you have for muscle contraction. This means you'll have a higher tolerance for heavier training

What to Watch For:
- Some people recommend taking 20 grams per day for 5 days, and then 5 grams per day after that... so it can get to be a lot
- It can cause the "creatine" bloat that some people experience making them look and feel stuffed
- It has been known to cause upset stomach and diarrhea in some people
- Low quality creatine might contain high amounts of dicyandiamide (a derivative of cyanide)
- Creatine may degrade to the substance creatinine. High levels of creatinine may be harmful to your health, so you want to be careful.

Where to Get Them

For the most part, if you look for supplements from top suppliers, you should be ok. As far as online sources, there are only two that I can recommend:

- GetProGrade.com: They are a refreshing trend in the supplement industry. These guys took a lot of time to create a different kind of supplement company. They get their supplements independently verified by a 3rd party laboratory to guarantee their honesty and integrity. They also have a customer service phone number, which is great because you have someone you can actually talk to. Also, I really like how informative their website is. They have tons of useful articles and tips on their site. I was turned on to them by fitness expert Shaun Hadsall and Shawn Lebrun, two highly trusted fitness experts that I relied on while writing this book.
- BioTrust.com: These guys also created a different kind of supplement company. Their main product is a high-quality, organic whey protein supplement that you can take after your workouts. I like them also because of their informative nature. If you get on their email list they send you tons of useful diet and nutrition information. It's always actionable and I actually go back to their

emails as reference material. They've obviously put a lot of effort into educating and even entertaining their customers. If you go and watch the video on their site you'll know what I mean. These guys were recommended to me by Craig Ballantyne, so I know they're legitimate. One of the owners of the company (Joel Marion) is a world renowned author and has written for lots of fitness websites.

So that's all I have to say about supplements. If I have anything else, I'll update this book and send it to my current customers.

Also, I will say that no supplement companies have paid me to promote them. However, I'm honest and I like honesty, so I'll tell you that if you buy anything from the links above, I'll get a small commission. It's not that much (won't even cover the cost of diapers for my 2 year old son) and it will NOT increase your purchase price. I've just worked out an arrangement where they give me a small commission for any customers that I refer to them. You're free to use those links, or to simply buy these supplements at your local health food store. It's totally up to you but these two companies have a solid reputation. .

Training Principle 1: Training for Strength vs. Training for Muscle Mass

One of the biggest myths I held to be true was that if you want to build muscle, you should lift heavy weights with low repetitions. And that if you want to "get cut" you should lift lighter weights with high repetitions. As you'll learn in this chapter, this couldn't be farther from the truth. In fact, it's the total opposite, and the ONLY way to "get cut" is to achieve low body-fat levels. Understanding the physiology of how a muscle gets bigger and stronger will help you achieve your goals.

Muscle is made up of tiny fibers, which contract to exert force. When you get strong, you actually increase the number of these muscle fibers. This is called myofibrillar hypertrophy. When you get larger muscles, you increase the fluid (sarcoplasm) in the actual muscle cell, this is called sarcoplasmic hypertrophy. This is why huge guys with big muscles aren't as strong as smaller power lifters.

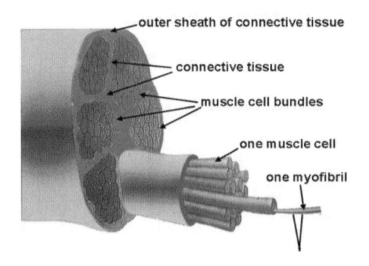

Training for Strength - Myofibrillar Hypertrophy

When you train for strength, you're training your body to be more efficient with the muscle it already has. Think of it like this, your muscles are made of different types of fibers. So when you lift a light weight, only a small amount of fibers are activated. The heavier the weight becomes, the more fibers get "recruited" into action. So if you curl a 10 pound weight, your nervous system will send a weak signal to tell your muscle to contract. Now if you lift a 100 pound weight over your head, your nervous system will send really strong signals to your shoulders, triceps, and lower back, "recruiting" them into action, Well, each time you recruit these fibers, you're telling your brain to send .stronger impulses to the muscles being worked. Over time, your nervous system is trained to utilize your muscles to exert the most amount of force possible. Training like this will get you defined muscles that are dense and strong.

Understanding this was an epiphany for me, because I never understood how skinny looking guys could bench nearly twice their body weight and dead lift almost 3 times their body weight. **Big muscles don't always equate to strength.**

Training your nervous system to become more efficient, means training it to fire strong impulses to your over and over again. You'll have to perform heavy lifts enough times to build a strong mind-to-muscle link. It is a skill that you must develop through practice over time.

Strength training requires you to lift heavy weights, for less repetitions. For example, if your bench press max is 150 lbs., lifting 140 lbs. five times will train your muscles to work harder. Over time, you'll notice dramatic increases in how much you can lift. So lifting heavy weights for low reps will get you strong. The only thing to remember is that this type of training is very taxing on your nervous system, so you want to get 4-5 minutes of rest between sets and you definitely don't want to do this type of training more than 3 times per week. When training for strength, none of your sets should be done to "failure". Doing this will cause your brain to send weaker impulses to your muscles, which means that your muscles will not contract as strongly, hurting your goal of gaining more strength.

Your reward will be strong muscles that are dense and angular like an Olympic gymnast.

Training for Mass - Sarcoplasmic Hypertrophy

Scientists aren't in complete agreement on how muscle actually grows, but most theories revolve around the idea that lifting weights breaks down muscles. Subsequently, muscles are thought to grow when the body rebuilds the muscle to protect itself from future stress.

Since muscles are thought to grow as a result of being "broken down", training for big, massive muscles requires the muscles to be under tension for longer periods of time than when training for strength. So "time under tension" is key to growing muscle. This is done by performing 8-12 repetitions of an exercise and working the muscle to near exhaustion. Overtime, this will damage the muscle and force it to repair itself. Part of the process is when the body rushes fluid to the muscle cells called sarcoplasm. The sarcoplasm increases the volume of the muscle cells, making them look larger. The increased volume makes the muscles look larger, without actually increasing strength. Of course, over time, the muscles will increase in size, but you shouldn't mistake a "pumped" muscle as a strong one. . At the cellular level, muscles grow when a mechanical load is placed they convert to an anabolic state, where they grow. The key to growth though is proper nutrition, water and rest. Eating adequate amounts of protein, carbohydrates, and fat will fuel the growth of the muscle and 7-9 hours of sleep per night allow your body to rebuild itself. Don't underestimate this, food, water, and rest are the main factors of gaining muscle. Your body is 70% water so even slight dehydration will affect your body's ability to build muscle. And since your body releases testosterone and growth hormone during sleep, you need to get rest if you want to get big. It's just that simple.

Be careful not to over train though. The ideal amount of time spent lifting weights is 30-45 minutes because this is the optimal time it takes for your body to release growth hormones (primarily testosterone). After this, your body could start releasing catabolic (muscle-destroying) hormones. This is helps explain why sprinters are so muscular and marathon runners are so thin.

So to gain muscle you want to perform an exercise 8-12 times per set and get plenty of food, water, and sleep so your muscles rebuild bigger and stronger versions of themselves.

This is because the micro trauma that exercise induces in the muscle stimulates protein synthesis, causing testosterone to be released and make the muscles grow. Lifting weight in the 8-12 repetition range causes more micro trauma in the muscle (time under tension) and greater hormone secretion.

Key Takeaways
- Strength is neurological because the nervous system is trained to send stronger impulses to the muscles, forcing them to "recruit" more muscle fibers and contract harder. You want to lift 2-6 reps of an exercise with a very heavy weight with 5 minutes of rest between sets. <u>Rest between sets is critical.</u>
- Gaining mass is caused by damaging your muscles by doing 8-12 reps of an exercise with a moderately heavy weight. This rep range ensures adequate "time under tension" so your muscles get sufficiently damaged. The muscles will fill with sarcoplasmic fluid (giving a "pumped up" look) and eventually as the muscles repair themselves, they will grow.
- Muscle and strength are built outside of the gym. Proper caloric and macronutrient intake is key (protein, carbs, and fat), as well as lots of water and 7-9 hours of sleep.
- The human body is extremely adaptable, so over time it will respond less to the stress placed upon it. The ideal workout program will combine both myofibrillar and sarcoplasmic growth by varying the number of repetitions and rest intervals between sets to build a strong physique and noticeable strength.

With all that said, there seems to be an inverse link between strength gains and muscle growth gains. Lifting heavy weights teaches the muscles to work better through neural adaptation, causing you to become stronger. However, your body will recruit less muscle fibers the more it adapts. The less muscle fiber you stimulate, the less you'll grow. That's why you have to vary your workouts to target both myofibrillar and sarcoplasmic hypertrophy, otherwise your body will adapt and you'll stop seeing results.

Training Principle 2: Fitness is Intensity Dependent, Not Time Dependent

Back in my martial arts days, lots of people would boast about how many years they spent studying. They thought somehow that training for lots of years meant that they were better than others. And I kind of thought the same thing. And then someone said something that made a lot of sense:

"It's not the years of kung fu, it's the kung fu in the years"

The same principle applies to working out. Lots of people spend hours on the gym, 6-7 times per week. Not only is that kind of schedule unsustainable for most busy guys (like you and me), it's not very productive. It doesn't matter if you train for 2 hours a day if most of the time is spent talking, waiting for machines, or flipping through your iPhone. People workout way too often with not enough intensity. The result is fatigue and burnout. You get stuck on a plateau and get discouraged that you don't see the results you want. As the quote above implies, it's not how long you're at the gym that counts, it's how you spend your time in the gym that matters. The key is to spend your limited amount of time exercising at the right level of intensity.

This book will show you how to optimize the results of your workout by doing each exercise with perfect form and maximum intensity - all in the least amount of time possible. Because after a certain point, your body doesn't respond to the stimulus placed upon it. Working out at a high intensity will help you cut down the time you spend in the gym, melt fat, and trigger fast growth in your muscles.

Getting a lean, ripped, athletic physique takes hard work and mental focus. Training with high intensity will forge the mental toughness and fortitude that many people need to tackle life's challenges.

So, intensity is one of the most important factors, but sadly, it's often missed or ignored in most fitness regimens and workout programs. To be perfectly blunt, performing any exercises or workout at a high intensity is extremely hard and requires a great level of focus which is why most people just don't do it. But since this product is about developing inner strength, fortitude, self-respect and confidence, that's exactly what you're looking for; a workout that requires you to develop clear and strong focus, so you can workout intensely and see the immense health benefits of doing so.

The benefits of working at a high intensity are greatly superior to that of longer, kind of low and slow type of moderate workouts. You know, I always like to say that, "Fitness is intensity-dependent and not time-dependent". So, although your workouts will be short, usually from 30 to 45 minutes at the max, they will be very productive workouts. As far as intensity, there are several variables that can increase the intensity of the workout. This includes the load or the amount of weight that you're using, how long you rest in between your sets and speed of doing the workout. So, any one of those variables can be tweaked and changed to increase or decrease the intensity of your workout, depending on your goals.

So, that being said, if you are not used to working at a high intensity, make sure that you start slow and start safe, get to know your body and your limits, and then gradually increase your intensity by either increasing the amount of weights that you're lifting, the time that you rest in between your sets or the speed with which you lift the weights. That's the best way to see steady, progressive gains and to prevent injury. As far as the definition of high intensity, you want to make sure that when you are working out, you are... I guess the easiest way to put it, is that when you're working out with high intensity, you'll feel it. You'll be huffing and puffing, breathing really hard, your face will become flush and you'll really feel that you've exerted yourself, and again, this will be part of developing your own self-respect and inner strength because you'll have a level of confidence and a level of self-respect for pushing yourself so hard.

So, again, when you're starting out, I recommend that you progressively build your intensity. You don't want to start too intensely and then end up injuring yourself or end up missing your workouts because you're too tired or you need too long to rest between workouts. So, it's better to start off with a moderate or lower level intensity when you first start and then to gradually and progressively work your way up once you've gotten the fundamentals and you understand how your body works. And again, with each workout, you do want to progressively increase the intensity, but again, I can't stress enough the importance of starting at a moderate and comfortable intensity at the beginning. This way you can keep your workout schedule to about three or maybe four days a week, and still keep it manageable with the current responsibilities of your busy life. As you'll learn in future chapters, circuit training or super-set style of working out is really helpful for creating a very intense workout, but at the same time, keeping it manageable and keeping it doable, especially with your busy schedule.

Try supersets or circuits will maximize the intensity of your workout. .

Training Principle 3: Compound Full-Body vs. Split Body Part Routines

This chapter is going to help you understand the differences between full body compound exercises and split body part workouts. Now, to be clear, full body workouts, where you're working out your entire body in the same day, will help you get that lean, muscular, defined athletic physique that most guys are looking for. But beyond just the aesthetics, it's going to give you the strength and the power to carry over in other aspects of your life as well, just giving you that edge in the rest of your life, as well as the self-confidence and self-respect that you're going to need to deal with all of life's obstacles. Part of the reason is that working out your entire body the same day forces your body to produce more hormones for growth, specifically growth hormone and testosterone which is beneficial for building muscle. It also helps you reduce the time that you spend in the gym. So when you work out your entire body with compound movements in the same day, you only really have to go to the gym three maybe four times a week, rather than going five or six times a week, which is not very practical for a lot of guys.

The Benefits of Compound, Full Body Workouts

Examples of compound exercises are exercises like the bench press, pull-ups, dips, push-ups, barbell rows, squats, lunges, dead lifts, and overhead presses. These are exercises that use compound movements and they require you to use more than one joint. So, with the bench press, for example, you're using your shoulder and your elbow. With squats, for example, you're using your knees and your hips. Compound movements are basically where you would use multiple muscle groups and multiple joints to perform one single action.

Another reason to do compound full body workouts is the results of the University of Wisconsin's study that found that guys that perform a full body workout involving the three big muscle exercises, (the bench press, power clean, and back squat) elevated their metabolisms for 39 hours after their workout. On top of that, they burned a greater percentage of their calories from fat during that time compared to guys who did not do a total body workout. So, for guys who want to get lean and get a defined muscular physique, completing intense full body workout with compound exercises three days a week is really the way to go. Of course, you're going to want to rest a day between your workout sessions, but during those rest days, your metabolism will still be in high gear, burning fat, even while you're not working out. On top of that, full body functional exercises stimulate your core so they help work your abs and your oblique's indirectly without you having to do endless sets of crunches, sit-ups and other boring ab exercises like that. .

As far as the benefits of full body compound exercises, they stimulate hormone growth. They stimulate the growth of testosterone and growth hormone, which helps you burn fat and build muscle primarily because the neuro-endocrine system is stimulated during these type of workouts. Doing compound full body workouts help to build a functional, athletic body. It just helps you get things done. Because your body is working as one functional unit, there's a great crossover into your life like athletics, self-defense and other types of sports because full body workout routines mimic the way your body naturally moves in real life, which is as a functional unit. Also, another benefit of a full body workout routine is that it targets all your muscle groups in every session.

On top of that, full body workout routines are great for beginners who are looking to lose weight or guys who are looking to build muscle as fast as possible. Because full body workouts stimulate so many muscles, you can expect a tremendous amount of muscle stimulation. You can expect a tremendous amount of growth hormone and testosterone to be secreted by your body, again, helping you burn fat and build muscle while keeping your time in the gym to a minimal.

Full body workouts also have a greater caloric expenditure per workout compared to split body part routines because literally hundreds of muscles are being worked and taxed in each session, requiring you to expend more energy, burn more calories, and of course, burn more fat in the process. So, again, it's really helpful for muscle growth. Another benefit of full body exercises is that it creates an incredible amount of micro-trauma, protein degradation and it depletes the glycogen storage of your body, leaving your body in an extremely prime state to soak up the nutrients and to promote anabolic growth, which is where your body is actually actively growing muscle, provided you give your body the proper nutrition of protein, carbohydrates, and fats to help it compensate for the intense workout that you've just performed.

Full body workouts comprised of compound exercises create a very functional, a very strong body that works as a unit, that prevents muscular imbalance and that promotes a functionally strong body. So if you look at the physiques of NFL running backs or wide receivers and even world-class sprinters, those athletes never train or almost never train with muscle isolation or with split body part workouts like just biceps, or just bicep curls, or just triceps extensions, or calf raises, or things like that. But even still, they are just lean, ripped, and extremely muscular.

The Benefits of Isolated, Split Body Part Workouts

So, while compound full body workout routines have a number of benefits, there are also benefits to split body part workouts. Those are where you're working out just one or two muscle groups per day, with only single joint exercises. So, for example, doing bicep curls and doing tricep extensions with calf raises. That would be one example of a body part split, where you're working certain muscles on one day, and then maybe another day, working another set of muscles with these isolated type of movements. One of the benefits to doing these split body part workouts is, because of the demanding nature of full body compound workouts, they're extremely fatiguing, which isn't really a good thing for lifts conducted near the end of your workout, so by the time you reach your compound movement number three and number four, you're suffering from just a high level of general fatigue so you're just tired, which makes your form a little bit sloppy.

Another benefit of split body part workout routines is that you get greater attention per muscle group. So, if on one day you're working out two muscle groups, like your biceps and your triceps, you don't have to worry about the rest of your body. You can focus all of your exercises for that day just in your biceps and your triceps, and do different variations of curls, tricep extensions, dips, things like that, that'll work those specific muscles that you're focusing on for that day. It results in more specific micro-trauma and more specific "damage" to those particular muscles, so that they grow faster. There's a more focused growth on those specific muscle groups when you're resting.

On top of that, split body part routines allow you to focus more attention on these specific muscles that you're working, so they're really ideal for bodybuilders and people who are concerned with building a very symmetrical physique, although it's not the best for building a functional solid physique. And then the third main benefit of split body part workouts are that, since full body part workouts are long and fatiguing, they sometimes have a tendency for trainees to overtrain. Whereas with a split based routine, you can get an intense, high quality workout in as little as a half an hour, just by focusing on the specific muscle groups that you're working that particular day. This also helps you focus better on your form, and again, it just helps you feel less exhausted at the end of your workout.

.

Key Takeaways

- So, the key takeaways are that full body compound exercises are excellent because they build a very well-rounded, solid physique, where the body is trained to work as a whole, making it extremely effective for training for sports like football, mixed martial arts, or boxing, or basketball, anything that requires you to move your entire body at the same time.

- It builds a very strong muscular physique because full body workouts will trigger hundreds of muscles across your body and it will trigger the greater production of growth hormone and testosterone, so it'll simultaneously help you burn fat and build muscle which is great for busy guys who don't have tons of time to create complex, elaborate workouts where one day is arms and back, and another day is chest and legs, and another day is another body part routine. So with a compound full body movements, you're able to get in and out of the gym in about 30 to 45 minutes, three times a week.

- Split body part routines allow you to focus more on specific muscle groups, reducing the risk of over-training and reducing the risk of having poor, sloppy form due to greater general fatigue.

- Split body part routines are great for bodybuilders or people who want to build large, symmetrical muscles.

- Split body part workout routines where you work out certain muscle groups on specific days is great especially if you have the time to work out five or six days a week. Whereas if you're really strapped for time and you want to build a really ripped, lean, functional physique like a sprinter, compound full body movements are definitely the way to go. .

Training Principle 4: The Science of Rest

Understanding rest intervals is extremely key if you want to get the most out of your workout. As you've learned in previous chapters, the intensity with which you work out controls the results that you get. The type of exercises that you choose, whether they're compound full body exercises versus split body part exercises, governs how your body will look and the type of training that you do, whether you're doing lower repetitions of heavier weights to build strength or higher repetitions of slightly less weights will force your body to increase muscle mass.

Rest is also another key factor in helping you define and sculpt the body that you want. Rest periods between sets are really an integral, but often overlooked contributor to the success of pretty much any workout program. So, the purpose of this chapter is to really help define rest and explain the importance of the rest during working out. Now when I speak about rest, I'm talking about the rest in between your sets during your actual workout, not the rest between one workout and the next, meaning between working out one day and then working out the next day. That's going be covered in a separate chapter. But here, we're going to focus our discussion just on the rest that's conducted between exercises of a workout on a specific day.

So, the rest period that you use during your workouts are defined by the type of workout and the type of goals that you're setting for yourself. So, for people who are almost absolutely concerned about strengths, you are typically going to work out using heavy, heavy weights, doing low repetitions, so you may be doing five repetitions of a weight that's about 90% of your one repetition, max. You don't really care about muscle hypertrophy, like sarcoplasmic hypertrophy, where you're building muscle and building mass, that's not your primary concern. So, for people who are concerned about strength like power lifters, and football players and exercises of that nature, your optimal rest period is going to be between three to five minutes.

One reason for this longer rest is to allow full phosphagen recovery before your next set. So, full recovery allows you to produce the greatest muscular force possible for each set that you perform and this will, over time, help you develop the greatest level of strength. Another good reason for a higher rest interval, meaning three to five minutes, is that when you're doing workouts with heavy loads or heavy weights, scientific research suggests that it produces greater testosterone levels, especially when you're using large compound exercises. And since you are producing higher levels of testosterone that should result in greater strengths. .

Also, if you recall from an earlier chapter, when you're training for strength, you're actually training your central nervous system to send stronger impulses to your muscles, forcing them to recruit more muscle fibers to lift the amount of weight that you're trying to lift. So, you do need a higher rest period for your central nervous system to refresh itself and prepare itself for the next heavy lift. As a general rule of thumb, the lower the repetitions and the heavier the weights, which is the range for strength training as we've discussed earlier, the longer you'll need to rest between your sets. So, if you don't rest long enough between your low repetition, heavy weight sets, your body will not be prepared to lift the next set which will make it harder for you to complete your full workout because your body is fatigued because it hasn't had enough time to replenish itself and prepare itself for the next heavy load.

Now, for people who are looking for hypertrophy or larger muscles, to build muscle mass and muscular endurance, your ideal rest period will be anywhere between 30 to 60 seconds. Another easy rule of thumb is that if you're working out to build muscle mass and increase your muscular endurance, you want to have a ratio of 1 to 1. Meaning you want to spend the same amount of time resting as you spent actually lifting weights. So, anyone who's looking to build muscle mass should try to have a rest of about 60 seconds, which is about the same amount of time that you'll be lifting the weights. Using this rest interval creates high lactate levels in your body in those specific muscles that are being exercised and this forces the body to improve its ability to deal with or to resist the accumulating lactate in your muscles.

So, over time, you'll get better muscular endurance. The more lactate there is in your muscles, the better your body becomes at protecting itself against the lactate, so over time, you'll get better muscular endurance. Also, these high volume, short rest period workouts have been also found to increase human growth hormone levels, when compared to training with just longer rest periods. So, as a rule of thumb for muscle hypertrophy, muscle growth and muscular endurance, the higher the repetitions and the lighter the weights, the shorter you want your rest periods to be.

Now the unique exception to this rule is circuit training. As you'll learn about later, circuit training generally involves more amounts of work and shorter periods of rest, and this is particularly helpful for increasing aerobic capacity and building muscular strength. The amount of muscular strength that you build with circuit training, which is where you'll do five or six exercises in a row, with maybe 30 seconds of rest in between, will be 30 to 50 percent less, so you'll gain less strength in doing circuit training, but it's particularly helpful for cardiovascular endurance and conditioning. So, in that case, you are lifting weights, but typically, they'll be lighter weights. You'll do five or six different exercises and then rest for about 30 seconds and then conduct the cycle all over again.

.

Key Takeaways

- Keep in mind that whatever your goals are for training, whether you want to build more strength or build more muscle. If you're a beginner, you'll need to rest more between your sets than someone who's been working out for a longer period of time. So, if you're just starting out, stay on the conservative side of your range and just listen to your body. There's a very fine line between an intense workout and exhausting yourself and possibly even injuring yourself, so you want to play it safe and decrease your rest intervals over time as you feel yourself getting stronger and you have more confidence in your body's ability to endure the higher intensity.
- Remember that changing the rest period is pretty much the same as changing the number of reps or the amount of weight that you lift, or even the number of sets that you perform of a specific exercise. So, it's an extremely important, but often overlooked part of your fitness routine. So, if you understand that by simply tweaking your rest intervals between exercises, you can help achieve your goals, whether it's to build strength or build muscle, you'll be much more apt to pay attention to the stopwatch.

- So, as far as the general recommendations, if you're doing heavier lifts of anywhere from one to five repetitions, you want to rest anywhere from three to five minutes. That's because you're training your central nervous system to recoup more muscle fibers and you need that time for your body to replenish itself, and again, that will trigger the strength gains or the mild fibular hypertrophy that we discussed earlier.
- Now if you're performing anywhere from eight to 12 repetitions of an exercise, your goal typically will be mass, or what's called "Sarcoplasmic Hypertrophy", where you're really trying to induce muscle growth. And in that situation, where you're performing eight to 12 reps of an exercise, you want to rest one to maybe two minutes maximum between your exercises.
- Remember that these are just guidelines, and again you're going to want to listen to your body, but as you become a more experienced lifter, you'll be paying more attention to your rest intervals, again depending on your specific goals.

So like we've learned in previous chapters, there's no one best way to work out, no one best type of workout routine, no one best type of rest interval. It really just depends on whether you intend to gain strength, gain muscle or get a leaner, slimmer physique. So again, just understanding the science of rest will definitely help you accomplish your goals.

Don't sacrifice results because you didn't pay attention to your stopwatch. Here's what Cosgrove recommends:

- 1 to 3 reps: Rest for to 5 minutes (strength - myofibrillar hypertrophy)
- 4 to 7 reps: Rest for 2 to 3 minutes (strength - myofibrillar hypertrophy)
- 8 to 12 reps: Rest for 1 to 2 minutes (mass - sarcoplasmic hypertrophy)
- 13 reps or more: Rest for 1 minute (mass - sarcoplasmic hypertrophy)

Like the fitness author, Craig Ballantyne likes to say, "***Make sure that you train hard, but safe, but hard.***" So hopefully, that helps to understand or helps explain the importance of rest intervals in between your workouts. .

Training Principle 5: The Only REAL Way to Get Abs

So, the common phrase is that, "Abs are made in the kitchen, not in the gym." That's so true, because a lot of guys try to work out their ab muscles because they want to get six packs, so they'll do exercises like crunches and sit-ups, thinking that that's going to help them the six pack that they desire. The thing they may not know, is that there's no way to spot-reduce fat in your body, so you can't target fat on your stomach or fat on your thighs, or fat on your arms, or fat under your chin. Really, the only way to lose fat is to work out your body and burn fat across your entire body.

Now, some people are more predisposed to accumulating fat on their hips and their waist, whereas other people are more predisposed to accumulating fat on their belly, but no matter where it tends to store itself on your body, the only way to get a ripped six pack is to focus on losing fat, reducing your body fat percentage, so that your ab muscles will naturally reveal themselves. So, you cannot spot-reduce fat, but you can spot-build muscle. So, whereas you cannot reduce fat exclusively on your belly or specifically on your thighs, you can build muscle on your thighs, you can build muscle on your shoulders, you can build muscle on your chest, etc.

But, unfortunately, losing fat does not work like that. As we discussed earlier, doing compound exercises with little rest in between, like circuit training, helps trigger your core muscles and inadvertently and indirectly conditions your abs without doing any sit ups or crunches. So, again, sit ups and crunches are definitely not the best way to reveal a strong, muscular, six-pack abdominal section.

So, contrary to popular belief, having six-pack abs does not mean that you have a strong core. It simply means that you have very little belly fat. In order for your core (mid-torso region) to be trained properly, you need to do full body exercises that force your core to stabilize the rest of your body. So, a great example of that would be back squats, or even front squats, where you're holding a barbell with a heavy weight across your back or across the front of your shoulders, and you do a squat. That forces your entire abdominal region to stabilize the rest of your body.

Another excellent exercise to trigger your core are planks, where you simply hold your body in push up position and just stay there. Side planks and other variations of planks are also just great exercises to work your core and to build stronger abdominal muscles, so that when you do lose the fat around your belly region, you'll be left with a strong and ripped six pack.

Just remember the purpose of your core and your torso muscles, and that is to provide greater stability and rigidity for the rest of your body to perform its other more functional movements. So, if you understand that, you'll realize why doing compound exercises like squats, like even a bench press, can help trigger and activate your core muscles. Or even exercises like push-ups will help you eventually, over time, as you shed belly fat, help you build a strong, ripped six pack that most guys want.

Sample Ab Workouts

Here are some great ab workouts you can do if you want to get six pack abs. Just remember, you have to get your body fat percentage down to 10% to 15% if you want to actually see your abs, so that's what you need to focus on first. But of course, working your abs isn't a bad thing before that. Just don't get frustrated if you don't see a six pack if you're over 15% body fat.

6-Pack Workout #1:
This workout came from Keith Lai at FitMole.com You can do this 2-3 times per week. Either after your cardio, or after lifting weights on your weight lifting days:

- Front plank for 2 minutes, rest 1 minute (basically remain in pushup position)
- Side plank for 2 minutes, rest 1 minute
- 3 sets of plank rows with a dumbbell (do a regular plank and lift the dumbbells of the ground, one arm at a time)

6-Pack Workout #2:
This one came from Greg O'Gallagher at Kinobody.com Same as above, you can do this 2-3 times per week. Either after your cardio, or after lifting weights on your weight lifting days:

- Hanging leg raises from a pull-up bar 10 – 15 times
- Hanging side-to-side knee ups 10-15 times
- 3 sets of plank rows with a dumbbell (do a regular plank and lift the dumbbells of the ground, one arm at a time)
- 2 sets of planks (as long as you can) .

Training Principle 6: Progressive Overload and Periodization for Progressive Gains

One of the other factors that, in addition to the rest intervals, the type of exercises you choose, and the number of repetitions that you lift as we've discussed in earlier chapters, is the actual load, or in other words, the actual weight you use when you are lifting weights. Whether you're trying to burn fat or build muscle, it's vital that you use an amount of weight that will challenge you. That being said, if you're not typically used to lifting heavy weights, you want to challenge yourself as much as safely allows. Again, like fitness expert Craig Ballantyne says, "Train hard. But Safe. But hard."

The concept of progressive loading means that you add more and more weight to the bar each time you work out. So every time you work out, you should be adding a little bit more weight to ensure that you are progressing properly and that your muscles are sufficiently stimulated to trigger more growth or to trigger greater fat loss. This is because your body is extremely smart and it adapts over time, so in order to get stronger, you have to always increase the weight or vary your exercise. This is because research shows that the better trained you become, the more your body's exercise efficiency "improves", meaning the same amount of activity burns fewer calories or triggers less muscle growth as time goes by.

This is really a simple concept. So, if you want to increase your strength and increase your body's ability to burn fat, a safe and steady goal is to add five pounds of weight to your workout every week. So, for example, if you bench 150 pounds this week, you want to make sure that the next time you are bench pressing, you add five pounds to the bar, and then five pounds to the bar after that, five pounds to the bar the time after that, and so on and so forth, ensuring that your body is always growing and doesn't plateau so the muscle growth or strength gains do not just stagnate.

If you find that you are reaching a plateau where you simply cannot gain more strength or you simply cannot add more weight to the bar, that's perfectly natural. Your body will naturally plateau at a certain point. We can't continue to grow muscle and gain strength forever. So, one creative solution to that problem is to vary your exercise; either vary the angle or vary the type of exercise that you're doing to help work out that particular muscle or your body from a particularly different angle. This forces your body to adapt and to grow, even though the weight may still be the same.

What's the Deal with "Muscle Confusion"?

Periodization is another technique to force your body to progress. This is basically where you cycle your workouts. For example, if you're accustomed to bench-pressing 170 pounds for 3 sets of 10 in every chest workout. Your periodized plan might look something like this:

Weeks 1-3
Three sets of 10 with 170 lb.

Weeks 4-6
Four sets of 5 with 195 lb.

Weeks 7-9
Three sets of 8 with 180 lb.

Weeks 10-12
Five sets of 4 with 185 lb.

The weight you lift and your repetitions progresses every three weeks. This produces more strength and size as the load on your muscles keeps increasing.

There are multiple types of periodization, but before we get to that, consider this:
Periodization allows you to take a set of movements (bench press, squat, deadlift, overhead press, and bent over row) and literally make an entire workout program that you can use for 6 to 12 months by simply changing the weight, repetitions, sets, and rest intervals you take. No need for any fancy or elaborate (a.k.a. dangerous) movements or equipment. As you can see, periodization workout is very scientific and sophisticated, yet it's extremely simple to do. It just boils down to manipulating the variables of your workout so your body constantly adapts.

.

Key Takeaways

- Remember that the only reason a muscle will get bigger or stronger is by increasing the amount of weight or the angle that that muscle has to work at. So since muscles respond to stress, I.e., lifting weights, they will progressively adapt and get progressively stronger to handle the stress that's being applied on them.

- If you want to increase your muscle growth and the amount of strength that you have, you have to constantly add weight to each one of your workouts every time you do work out. This will force your body to progressively build muscle and progressively grow stronger.

- The goal is to stimulate, not annihilate your muscles. So, that's why we choose a safe weight of five extra pounds per workout, so that your body is forced to grow but it's done in a safe, and controlled, and sustainable fashion because the last thing you want to do is overexert yourself and not work out for two weeks which will, of course, negate any of the strength and muscle growth improvements you've made.

- Another way to progressively overload your muscles is to simply cycle your workouts. So, for example, if you're doing a bench press of 150 pounds, the next time you work out, you can do an incline bench press of 150 pounds. And then the next time you work out you can do dumbbell bench press where you have two 75-pound dumbbells and perform a bench press with those two exercises. So again, you are progressively challenging your body, not by adding more weight but by simply varying the exercise that you do, again, giving your body another reason to stimulate muscle growth. .

Training Principle 7: The "Supreme 7" Movements to Build Muscle, and Lose Fat

The biggest factor for busy guys not working out is that they feel their workouts are too complex, too hard to keep up with, too hard to maintain, hence, they're not able to sustain their workout schedule. So, this chapter is really, like the rest of the book, designed to show you seven simple movements that you need to do in order to build the strong, ripped, lean, muscular, functional body that most guys want. I mean, after all, that's why guys read magazines like Men's Health and Men's Fitness, because they love the way the cover models look and they want to build a body just like theirs. So in order to do that, especially if you're a busy guy with a wife and kids and a demanding career and extracurricular activities that you do, you need to simplify it. So, this chapter will explain the Supreme Seven Movements, as well as their variations. And once you understand these movements and their variations, you'll be able to develop and craft a very solid and a very helpful workout routine that will help you, as I mentioned, burn fat and build muscle.

These movements and their variations will help build a lean muscular physique that athletes like sprinters have. Later, we're going to use these seven exercises and their variations to engineer a full body workout that uses these compound movements to build functional strength and trigger muscle growth.

One thing that Arnold Schwarzenegger used to say, and again if you remember, Arnold Schwarzenegger, in addition to being an actor and the former Governor of California, had a background of being Mr. Olympia and he actually won Mr. Olympia seven times. And he was once asked why his arms are so big and what he did to train his arms, and he actually said that he used to squat and everyone laughed at him because they thought, "How can squats increase the size of your arms?" But research later came out, proving that what Arnold Schwarzenegger said was actually true.

So, that proved the effectiveness of these seven simple exercises. You don't need to have lists of hundreds and hundreds of exercises that are really complex and complicated and difficult to do. These seven exercises and their variations can be done at nearly any gym in the world, requiring you to only use really one or two pieces of equipment. So again, you can get that goal of working out three times a week, about 30 to 40 minutes per workout. These exercises are: .

1. **Squat:**
    - Front squat
    - Overhead squat
    - Box squat
    - Dumbbell/Kettlebell squat
    - Lunges (dumbbell or barbell)
2. **Overhead Press:**
    - Barbell/Kettlebell
    - Military
    - Behind/Front of Body
    - Push Press
    - One-arm
    - Alternating
3. **Deadlift:**
    - Conventional
    - Snatch Grip
4. **Bench Press:**
    - Wide/Medium/Close Grips
    - Reverse grip
    - Incline/decline
    - Dumbbell/Kettlebell
    - Push-up Variations
    - Dips

5. Upper Body Pulling:
- Chin-up/Pull-up Variations
- Cable Rowing
- Barbell/Dumbbell/Kettlebell Rows
- Renegade Rows

6. Clean and Jerk:
- Power Clean
- Dumbbell/Kettlebell Clean
- Dumbbell/Kettlebell Jerk and combinations of the two together

7. Snatch:
- Hang Snatch
- Dumbbell/Kettlebell Snatch
- One-arm Barbell Snatch

·

Bilateral vs. Unilateral Movements

These are all great movements and you should use them, but one thing to keep in mind is to focus on unilateral movements. That means movements that you need to do movements that require you to use your limbs independently. For example, if you only do bench presses and rows with barbells, your stronger limb is mostly likely bearing most of the weight. Doing unilateral exercises on the other hand elicit more core function due to the instability in the load. Doing unilateral exercises is very functional and mimics actions you do in real life like lifting grocery bags, carrying your kids, throwing a football, etc. The added benefit of unilateral movements is that they make your bilateral movements stronger. Quick tip, all you have to do is do movements with dumbbells rather than a barbell. Here are a few examples of unilateral movements:

- Dumbbell rows
- Dumbbell bench press
- Lunges
- Dumbbell overhead press
- One-arm dumbbell snatch
- Dumbbell clean and press
- Etc.

With these exercises, each limb is forced to work by itself. This forces your core to stabilize your body, leading to a better and stronger mid-section making it easier to get a 6-pack. .

Training Principle 8: Strength Circuits to Build Muscle and Burn Fat

So, in the previous chapters we've talked about the differences between building strength and building muscle mass, which is primarily, the number of repetitions and the amount of weight that you're using. We talked about intensity and how heavy and how fast you're lifting the weights. We talked about the differences between compound movements that work out your full body versus split body part routines, and we talked about the importance of rest intervals between your sets to help build your lean muscular physique.

In this chapter, we're going to talk about putting all those factors together to really practically burn fat and build muscle. So, the assertion that I'm going to make is that especially for busy guys who don't have five or six days a week to spend in a gym, performing functional, full-body, weight-bearing exercises in a high-intensity method, like supersets or circuit training, is the single most effective way to develop a lean muscular build and to literally burn and melt fat from your body.

A lot of people equate circuit training or superset type of training with light weights or with conditioning or just merely fat loss, but this is definitely not the case. Strength training coach Zach Even-Esh, if you know anything about him, he runs the Underground Strength Camp website, will attest that he does use circuit training frequently and with heavy weights in his own workouts, and it definitely does pack on muscle and strength. However, it's extremely difficult to do and it requires you to prepare for the intense focus and physical demands that this type of workout will place on your body. But again, for busy guys who want to build a really ripped, strong, functional physique, as well as the inner strength, the mental fortitude, and the self-respect that you will build in the process, this is really the best and the ideal type of workout.

History

As far as the history of traditional strength training and muscle building, traditionally, strength training was performed in separate blocks. So, for example, someone might run in the morning and then do gymnastics or some type of resistance training in the afternoon, or even alternate between days such as performing strength exercises on Monday, Wednesday and

Friday, and then running on Tuesday, Thursday and Saturday, etc. Also, traditional strength training is when all of the repetitions of a particular exercise are completed before moving on to the next exercise. This is referred to as "station training". Basically this type of training is ideal for complex movements like Olympic lifts. So, for example, an Olympic lifter might perform 3 sets of dumbbell snatches, followed by 3 sets of clean and jerks, followed by 3 sets of squats. Or a typical bodybuilder might do 3 sets of the bench press, 3 sets of squats and then 3 sets of rows, just basically performing 3 sets of each exercise and then moving on to the next exercise.

Now, circuit training or super-setting exercises on the other hand is slightly different. It's where you perform three or four, sometimes up to six different exercises in a row, with no rest in between. So, for example, you might do:

- a set of push-ups for 30 seconds,
- a set of dips for 30 seconds,
- a set of squats for 30 seconds,
- a set of overhead presses for 30 seconds
- and then lastly, followed by maybe jumping jacks for 30 seconds.

This type of training can be used effectively for both building strength and building muscle, but really, the selling point of this type of training or this circuit training where you're doing multiple weight bearing exercises in a row, is to burn fat while you're lifting the weights. You're not necessarily lifting for strength or mass, you're lifting to create a human growth hormone response where your body secretes more of this human growth hormone, which will help you burn a significant amount of body fat. Doing this as a high-intensity circuit training with weights, done properly, will keep your heart rate up, and since you're using heavy weights or moderately heavy weights, you will be preserving muscle mass in the process.

Now, to be clear, these workouts, when done properly, with good form and done one right after another, with maybe one minute of rest in between each of these sets of six exercises, is extremely difficult and it will help you develop an element of mental toughness and confidence as you push through the discomfort and the intensity of these exercises. You will definitely see your body transform, both in seeing the fat in your body start to diminish, as well as increased muscular definition. And when you're at the gym working out like this, you definitely will get stares from other people at the gym who look at you and admire the intensity and the seriousness with which you're taking your workout. And you'll strangely start to notice how other people are maybe wasting time or maybe not working out as efficiently on their workouts as you are.

When you're doing a circuit training type of workout with heavy weights, your time in the gym will be very efficient and very well-used. So you won't have time to chat up the ladies, to flip through fitness magazines, or to play with your iPhone. You're going to be there at the gym for one reason, and one reason only, and that's to work!

As far as the research behind the effectiveness of these circuit training workouts, Ball State University researchers discovered that fat-burning hormones increased with completing even just one set of a circuit. So for example, doing these six exercises, like I mentioned, could really help increase your body's ability to burn fat.

Also, by closely adhering to the specific rest periods of no longer than, about 75 seconds to 90 seconds in between these circuits, you're further speeding fat loss. That's because during your circuit, you're accumulating the chemical called "lactate" in your bloodstream, and high lactate levels are typically associated with elevated levels of fat-burning hormones. But the reason you want to keep your rest intervals short in between these sets is if you rest too long between sets, the oxygen that you breathe in will help your body clear the lactate from your bloodstream. However, if you keep your recovery time short, you'll have higher levels of lactate and fat-burning hormones in your bloodstream, causing your body to burn fat even while you're at rest.

So, in circuit training, where you're performing multiple exercises in a row of about six to eight reps, is great for, as I mentioned, burning fat and building muscle at the same time. Although, not the most effective way to build the most amount of muscle or the most amount of strength because it's still primarily an aerobic workout, using weights for additional resistance.

Supersets for Super Gains
Now, if you want the best of both worlds, super-setting or doing tri-sets, is even a more effective way of getting the cardiovascular benefits of circuit training, as well as the strength and muscle mass gaining benefits of doing a traditional strength and muscle-building workout.

When you perform supersets, you're combining two or sometimes even three exercises in a row. The exercises have to be structured in such a way that they work separate muscle groups, so as not to induce unnecessary fatigue in your muscles. So, an ideal superset would be:

- 8 squats followed immediately by
- 8 bench presses followed immediately by
- 8 barbell rows

You would rest for 1-2 minutes and then do the same thing all over again.

You typically want to be at about 85% of your one rep maximum. So for example, if you can squat 200 pounds as your max, you want to be somewhere around 160 pounds, so you want to do a squat of about 160 pounds, six to eight times, followed immediately by a bench press. So, if your bench press max is 200 pounds, you want to do about six to eight reps of a bench press, and if your barbell row maximum is 200 pounds, you want to do 150 pounds of barbell rows, six to eight times, and then you rest for one to two minutes.

This type of training gives you the cardiovascular benefits of circuit training, but because of the heavier weights that you're using, and the fact that the weights or the movements that are being used work out different muscle groups, it allows your body to lift these heavier weights without experiencing specific fatigue in the muscles. So when you're doing your squats, you're working out your legs and your core. When you do your bench press, you're working out your shoulders, your triceps, and your chest. And when you do your barbell rows, you're working out your biceps, and your shoulders, and your back primarily, during that particular exercise. So although your heart rate will be up, and your body will be producing higher amounts of testosterone and growth hormones, your muscles are not to the point of collapse, where you're experiencing specific muscle fatigue in each one of those muscles.

Key Takeaways

- Use circuit training to blend the information that we learned in the previous chapters which is the proper amount of weight and repetitions to trigger either greater strength or muscle growth, the appropriate intensity at which you should be working out at, the types of exercises that you do, whether they're compound exercises that work the entire body or they're split, more isolated type of exercises, and of course, the rest intervals in between the sets of your workout. So, lifting heavy weights, using your entire body to lift heavy weights, of two or three exercises in a short period of time, increasing the rate at which your body breaks down and rebuilds protein, this metabolism boost will last up to 48 hours after you've finished lifting.

- To take the circuit training concept to an even further level, you want to use what's known as "supersets," where you're using alternating muscle groups, two or three exercises that use alternating muscle groups that cause greater general fatigue, causing your heart rate to be elevated, but without causing the specific muscle fatigue of working out a specific muscle group too much. So, the example of that would be to do squats, followed by bench press, followed by barbell rows, or another alternative would be squats, followed by overhead press, followed by dead lifts.

- These supersets are a great technique for increasing muscle size because it boosts the release of anabolic hormones of testosterone and growth hormone, which is again, responsible for building muscle and burning fat, respectively. And of course, it reduce the amount of time that you spend at the gym, as well as the number of machines and the amount of equipment that you use. So, you're able to get a very efficient, very, very productive workout, in a very, very small amount of time. .

- Varying the rest intervals between your supersets will help you increase the intensity. Over time, you're going to reduce the rest intervals in between your sets. Or you can add weights, again, to modify the intensity and to help with your goals, whether they'd be adding more muscle mass, gaining more strength or burning more fat. .

Training Principle 9: High Intensity Interval Training for Fat Loss

Sprinting is critical to building a lean, athletic body. Just compare a marathon runner to a sprinter and you'll see the difference in physique. We're going to use the same principles to build a lean, muscular body.

Compared to "steady state" cardio where you jog, or bike, or swim at a constant pace for 30-45 minutes, interval training, which is characterized by one minute of intense activity followed by a minute of lower intensity activity has been shown to burn fat and maintain muscle mass. Let's take a look at the science of why interval training (in the form of sprints) is a great way for busy guys to burn fat and maintain muscle to build a lean, ripped physique.

The Science of Interval Training

Interval training causes muscles to adapt differently than "steady state" cardio because it requires your body to use anaerobic energy systems, meaning you use up the glycogen (stored carbs) in your muscles faster than with traditional "steady state" cardio. This type of training also causes your body to release growth hormone, which helps burn fat, making it ideal for guys who are lifting weights to build more muscle and strength while shedding body fat at the same time.

As far as increasing overall health of your heart and lungs, this is done by improving the delivery of oxygen to your heart and lungs as well as how that oxygen is used by your body. Increasing the efficiency of these two factors leads to not only a ripped physique, but a strong, healthy heart. Because of this efficiency, trainees typically need to train less than if they were doing "steady state" cardio.

So because interval training works your aerobic and anaerobic systems, your anaerobic system will uses energy stored your muscles (glycogen aka carbs) for these short, but intense bursts of activity. Your anaerobic metabolism works without oxygen, and the by-product of that work is lactic acid. As lactic acid builds in your body, it creates a state of "oxygen debt" in your body. During recovery periods, your heart and lungs work together to "pay back" this oxygen debt, helping to break down the lactic acid. In this way, your aerobic system uses oxygen to convert carbohydrates to energy. Over time, this is how your body becomes more efficient at delivering oxygen to your muscles, as well as becoming more efficient at compensating for the "oxygen debt" by using oxygen to turn carbohydrates into energy.

So interval training (aka sprinting) gets you lean and in shape fast by improving oxygen utilization at the muscular level.

The "Afterburn Effect" Explained

The "afterburn effect" has become really popular these days. It refers to the amount of calories your body burns after your workout. As described earlier, it has to do with how oxygen is consumed both during and after your workout. The 2 main key factors to burning calories during your workout are:

- **Calories Burned During Exercise (O2)** - This is the number of calories you burn during your workout. This is measured because the amount of oxygen uptake (the amount your body uses) is proportional to the number of calories burned
- **Calories Burned AFTER Exercise (EPOC)** – As discussed above, at higher workout intensities, your body builds an "oxygen debt" because you're working out so hard. Then EPOC (excess post-exercise oxygen consumption) So the "afterburn effect" is when your body makes up for this debt, which burns calories for up to 48 hours after the high intensity activity

How to Perform Intervals

Interval training is usually done with sprints, on a stationary bike, running stairs, or with body weight movements, however, most studies of interval training are done with trainees on a stationary bike. Stationary bikes are recommended for beginners who aren't used to running as well.

Interval training will improve your metabolic performance, and will help you burn calories up to 48 hours after your workout. The cool thing about interval training is that it's based on time rather than distance. So rather than running a certain number of miles, you perform intense activity for alternating periods of work and rest. An added benefit of working based on time is that you develop an iron will and a sense of mental toughness:

- 3 to 5 minute warm up
- intense running for 1 minute
- low intensity for 1 minute
- repeat 5-6 times

Suffice it to say, if you want to get lean and ripped, you have to sprint. That's because as your body burns fat, it could potentially burn muscle as well. Lifting weights and sprinting is critical to ensuring that your body burns fat and maintains muscle. Here are other exercises you can do in an interval style of high intensity/low intensity:

- Running Stairs
- Jumping Rope
- Hill Sprints
- Jumping Exercises (box jumps, squat jumps, etc.)

The key to making intervals work is the "interval" part where you switch between the two extremes of intense activity and rest, otherwise you're doing a regular "steady state" cardio workout. If you don't rest between the intervals you won't be able to sustain the intensity and subsequently won't get the benefits.

There is no one best way to perform intervals, just start slow and progressively increase intensity. This will help trigger the famed "afterburn effect" where your body burns calories for up to 48 hours after exercise.

Key Takeaways

- Low intensity "steady state" cardio burns calories while the activity is being performed

- Short, high-intensity interval training has been proved to burn calories for up to 48 hours after working out; meaning you can burn calories doing nothing

- Anaerobic (strength training) workouts increase the Excess Post-exercise Oxygen Consumption, where your muscles accumulate an "oxygen debt", which is then compensated for, allowing your body to turn glycogen into energy

- Intervals can be done with any type of exercise; it's just characterized by 60 seconds of intense effort, and 60 seconds of moderate effort for 5-6 rounds.

Training Principle 10: Developing Power

Part of building a strong, functional physique is to build power. Power is the ability to perform a specified amount of work in the shortest time possible. Things like throwing a punch, kicking a soccer ball, and swinging a golf club all require power. So the difference between power and strength is the ability to exert a maximum amount of force within a specified amount of time, whereas strength is the ability to exert maximal force with no concern about time.

If you're training for sports, the best way to develop power for your sport is to practice that sport. So if you're an MMA fighter that wants to build more powerful punches, you'll want to throw punches, same goes if you want to improve your golf swing. As far as building general power, that is done best with Olympic style lifts like the snatch, power clean, and split jerk. Now these are highly technical lifts and should be done with proper form and moderate weight until you build proper strength levels.

To develop power in the gym, you want to recruit as many motor units as possible. This means doing actions explosively, so that the rate of force is increased. Of course, the greater the strength, the greater power you will have, so it's crucial to work on building strength with heavier loads, and then lightening the load and focusing on speed progressively. Given that the greater the strength, the more power we can develop, it is crucial that strength be developed first with heavier loads, then the load lightened and the speed of contraction be increased progressively. However, once we have developed strength and then start developing power (speed-strength), we must continue to maintain strength by 1-2 sessions per week of strength training.

As mentioned earlier, this can be done in a number of ways... you don't just want to lift a weight, you want to focus on explosively lifting it, while maintaining control. This has the greatest effect on developing power, building endurance, and boosting your metabolism. In addition to Olympic movements like squats, clean and jerks, and snatches, you can use exercises like bodyweight squat jumps and dumbbell squat presses.

3 Benefits of Lifting Explosively

Fitness expert Chad Waterbury wrote an excellent article where he discussed this topic. He mentioned a study done of two different groups of men, everything was the same about them except the speed they used to lift the weight. Here's the breakdown:

Slow Group
Exercise: Squat
Sets: 4
Reps: 8
Load: 60% of 1 rep max (1RM)
Rest: 90 seconds
Tempo: two seconds down, two seconds up

Explosive Group
Exercise: Squat
Sets: 4
Reps: 8
Load: 60% of 1 rep max (1RM)
Rest: 90 seconds
Tempo: two seconds down, lift up as fast as possible

The results from the research concluded:

"Explosive concentric muscle contractions may be more effective than slow contractions for

enhancing energy-expenditure responses for weight loss when using resistance exercise"

That means that the group that lifted explosively burned more fat than those that had a slower tempo, that's despite lower levels of lactate found in the muscle.

Also, lifting explosively recruits more muscle groups. For example, doing an overhead press works your shoulders and lower back. But doing it explosively works your abs because they are forced to stabilize your body against the rapid release of force. This recruitment of additional muscle allows you to lift heavier loads as well.

Lastly, lifting explosively allows you to build "strength endurance". For example, if you're a sprinter that runs a 400 meter dash in one minute, you'll want to explosively do squats for about one minute (the same time it takes to do the run) so you're not only building real strength, the strength training done with endurance in mind will have a crossover effecting in your actual sport.

Bottom line: lift explosively to get stronger, burn more fat, and to have crossover in real life. .

Training Principle 11: Cut THEN Bulk?

Traditional wisdom among bodybuilders is go in the "bulk" phase to build muscle and then the "cut" phase to look defined and lean. Busy guys who want to lose weight can't really do that. For guys like us, it's smarter to get eat sensibly and workout to get lean and strong... and then once you look the way you want, then you can strategically add muscle mass. But it all comes down to you and your goals. Remember, everything works - but nothing works forever.

If you're thin and want to build muscle, then you should train for muscle growth and eat a slight caloric surplus. If you're overweight then focus on losing weight and cutting the fat with your diet and a smart training protocol that enhances the "afterburn" effect. So if you're a younger 135 lb. guy, newer to weight lifting, with a faster metabolism, then of course you're going to want to bulk because you'll have something to show for your efforts. But if you're older, a little heavier, don't have lots of time, want to get lean and muscular, you'll want to take a more progressive approach to steadily lose fat and get a more muscular physique then you should cut the fat and then strategically bulk.

There is no one best method. Just pick one and make it happen.

Pro and advanced bodybuilders usually benefit from bulking cutting but in my opinion, beginners and intermediates do not. The last thing an overweight beginner should focus on is bulking up. They should focus on body composition (fat loss) through diet and an effective workout program.

At the end of the day, it's up to you. Some people like bodybuilders will bulk up on muscle and then cut their weight with cardio and aggressive dieting. But for guys like you and me, it may be a good idea to focus on eating healthy, working out intensely (cardio and weight lifting) so you get lean and muscular, and then focusing on building muscle if you so desire. .

Training Principle 12:
The Science of Warming Up

Warming up is one of the most important things you can do for your body before a workout. This is so important for so many reasons, yet many guys ignore it, or just don't do it right.

Think about it this way; your workout is like remodeling your kitchen. There's a lot of demolition. You can't just start jack hammering your kitchen floor, breaking down your cabinets with a sledge hammer, and swinging an axe through your walls before preparing the rest of your house for the mayhem. So why should working out be any different? The truth is, lifting weights is taxing on your body. They prevent injury, promote circulation, help you lift more weight, loosen ligaments and tendons, and generally prepare your body for the workout. On top of that, properly warming up will make your actual workout feel so much easier.

Pro athletes understand the importance of warming up. Just look at what professional basketball players and Major League Baseball pitchers do before a game. So hopefully you're convinced to spend the few extra minutes it takes to warm up properly.

How to Warm Up

A lot of guys think they can do a few arm circles and some stretching and jump right into lifting weights. Others may spend a few minutes on a treadmill or stationary bike. Here's a quick run-down of each kind:

General Warmups: This includes running on a treadmill or riding on a stationary bike for a few minutes. You can even perform air squats, lunges, and pushups. This is good because it's low intensity and will get your blood flowing, eliminate the cracks from your joints by promoting the spread of synovial fluid, which helps lubricate your joints and prevent friction.

Specific Warmups: This includes doing the exact exercise that you'll be doing, at a lower weight/intensity. For example, if you're squatting 225lbs, you want to progressively work your way up to your work weight by starting with an empty bar and adding 25lbs to 45 lbs. each time until you reach your work weight. It would look like this:
. -Empty Bar (45lbs) x 5
-95 lbs. x 5
-135lbs x 3
-185lbs x 2
-225lbs x however many reps you normally do

Specific warm ups allow you to focus on your form gradually and progressively. Also, even though you're adding weight, since you're decreasing the repetitions, you won't feel exhausted once it's time to perform your actual workset. This is a great way to not only make your actual workout feel easier, but to make sure that you're performing your lifts properly so you don't hurt yourself.

You particularly want to follow this warmup scheme if you're lifting heavy weights or big, compound movements like squats, deadlifts, bench presses, etc.

A Quick Word on Stretching

Contrary to popular belief, stretching before a workout isn't the best thing. There is not enough scientific evidence to prove that stretching before working out prevents injury. Popular Mechanics Magazine reported that researchers from Florida State University concluded that stretching before running makes runners 5% less efficient, meaning that they had to burn more energy to run at the same pace. That same article talked about Italian researchers who found that stretching (touching your toes) change how your muscles generate and transmit force as well as alter the signals that the brain sends to your muscles.

In other words, there's nothing wrong with stretching after you work out, just make sure that you don't skip a warm up before your workout.

Training Principle 13: The Science of the "Deload Week"

Let's say you've been working out for a few months. You're lifting heavier weights, for more repetitions and you're seeing noticeable changes in your physique. Awesome. Since you've been lifting for a few months, you're noticeably stronger. So you're in the gym again, getting ready to squat more than you ever have, and you notice your knee buckling in a bit. After your workout, you feel a strain on the inside and outside of your right knee. All of a sudden you're limping around, worried that you tore a ligament in your knee. You take a week off from the gym and start researching the importance of taking a break. Lesson learned.

That's exactly what happened to me… and I don't want it to happen to you.

You Don't Get Stronger In the Gym

One of the biggest things most guys ignore when working out is the importance of taking a break. Here's the rub; you don't get bigger and stronger when you work out. You break your body down so that it can repair and rebuild itself. That's when you get bigger and stronger. Seems pretty innocuous, but it's so important to getting leaner, stronger, and more muscular that I had to share my personal story above to make sure you don't make the same mistake.

What's a "Deload Week"?
You do this by incorporating a "deload week" into your workout program. That means that you don't lift weights for an entire week. This allows you to rest your body, repair your muscles, allow your joints and connective tissue (ligaments and tendons) to heal, etc. The thing is that although you should be only lifting weights every other day, that's not enough rest. You need to factor in a one week "deload" where you don't lift any weights to give your joints a chance to heal. This is because your muscles and your joints don't operate on the same timeline. In other words, just because you don't feel soreness in your muscles doesn't mean you don't need a break. Since your joints operate on their own schedule, you need to factor in rest time to keep them healthy and injury free.

Don't be all macho and think you can skip this. A deload week is not a sign of chickening out or weakness. It's an intelligent, calculated, and highly-crucial part of your workout program.

How To Do It

Factoring a deload week into your training routine is really easy. Most serious lifters will tell you that the ideal deload schedule is to lift heavy for 3 weeks and then take 1 week off. If you do mostly bodyweight exercises or circuits with light weights, deloading won't be as important. In this case, you'd just lift 40% of your regular reps at 50% of your one-repetition max for about 5 repetitions. But if you're lifting heavy weights in big, compound movements like squats, deadlifts, bench presses, overhead presses, and bent over rows, you'll really benefit from lifting for 3 weeks and then taking one entire week off. It's important to stay consistent with this and not take it for granted.

If you're lifting serious weights (70% of your one-repetition max or higher) you should take a deload every 3 weeks. Others might be able to take it every 6 weeks or so.

During this time you can still stay active and do things you like such as playing golf, swimming, biking, hiking, walking, etc. Just don't lift weights so your joints, ligaments, and tendons have a chance to recuperate. So you don't have to give up being active, just stop lifting weights.

Don't Worry: You Won't Lose Your Muscle

Also, some people are afraid that taking time off will cause them to lose their strength, but this isn't really true. A recent study concluded that it takes about 3 weeks to lose strength. The researchers took 2 groups of trainees: one group worked out consistently for 15 weeks, the other worked out for 6 weeks, then took 3 weeks off, then worked out for 6 weeks, then took 3 weeks off again. Amazingly, both groups progressed in terms of muscle growth and strength gains. This is given the fact that the second group didn't do anything for 3 weeks at a time!

On top of that, the second group did not lose muscle mass.

Now, during those 3 weeks, you may lose some strength, but if you remember from Training Principle 1, strength is more neurological than muscular. So even though you can lose strength in less than 3 weeks, you will quickly gain it back once you start lifting weights again, you will "reignite" those neural pathways and quickly gain your strength back.

3 Things to Get Right - Sleep, Water, and Stress Management

So we've covered the proper rep range and rest intervals for muscle growth vs. muscle strength, we discussed the difference between compound exercises vs. split body part routines, training intensity, the importance of progressive overload so your body keeps getting stronger, and the importance of interval training. You would think that this is what really causes your body to build muscle and burn fat... but that's only partially true.

The real growth and repair your body experiences is when you're NOT in the gym. That's because working out simply stimulates the muscles to grow, whereas during rest they have the ability to repair themselves. That means, there is a point of diminishing returns where working out too long simply brings you no benefit. That's why it's critical to focus on working out intensely when you're in the gym and getting proper rest and nutrition during your off days.

Your body creates a few hormones that in addition to other things, help you build muscle and burn fat. Understanding how to utilize will help you get the body you want. Here's a quick breakdown:

TESTOSTERONE

Testosterone is a hormone found in both men and women. It's probably the most well-known of all hormones and regulates lots of critical functions like libido, energy, bone health, immune function and muscular development. It is created when special cells in your testicles convert cholesterol into testosterone. It's then released into your body and has been found to peak in the morning.

GROWTH HORMONE

We've discussed this hormone a lot throughout the book. It's created by your pituitary gland and is secreted the most at night, and then in small 4 hour increments after that. Once growth hormone enters your system, it helps improve your metabolism, glycogen production, and protein synthesis. This is a critical hormone to getting lean and ripped, and training the proper way (intense cardio and compound lifts) will elicit the best production of this critical hormone.

Here's How to Engineer Your Hormones So You Get Ripped

So you want your body to produce testosterone and growth hormone, as well as to use insulin to shuttle glucose and nutrients to your muscles.

And you want to make sure that your body doesn't unnecessarily secrete cortisol, because it is really counter-productive if you want to burn fat and build muscle. Here's how to regulate these hormones:

1). Shorten Workout Time: You want to make sure that you only workout for 30-60 minutes at a time. This is because working out more than that will trigger the production of higher levels of cortisol. When that happens, your body starts to convert muscle into fuel. Now unless you're using steroids to counteract the negative effects of cortisol, make sure that you spend a good, quality 30-60 minutes in the gym and no more.

2). Get Rest Between Workouts: I've said it earlier, and it's true that you want to stimulate, not annihilate your muscles when you work out. So you need at least a day of rest in between workouts to allow your body to rebuild muscle tissue that was damaged while lifting weights. If you work out too much or for too long, your body will start to produce cortisol, and we already know how detrimental that can be.

3). Get 7-9 Hours of Sleep: Sleep is probably one of the most underestimated factors in losing fat and building muscle. Sleep is when your body creates growth hormone. Lots of guys think they can stay up late and function well on 5 hours of sleep. To ensure that you're in an anabolic (muscle building) state, getting enough sleep is essential. The more you sleep, the more growth hormone you produce. On top of that, not enough sleep triggers the stress hormone cortisol, which will make it hard to lose weight and build muscle and lower testosterone levels.

Getting certain nutrients in your diet are associated with better sleep patterns. These include vitamin C, lycopene, and selenium. They can be found in the following foods:

Lycopene: This cancer-fighting antioxidant can be found in tomatoes, watermelon, and pink grapefruit.

Vitamin C: Just a cup of strawberries or one kiwi packs over 100% of your daily value of this heart and cancer-protective antioxidant.

Selenium: One ounce of Brazil nuts or a can of tuna are both great sources of this that's key for healthy immune function.

4). Drink Lots of Water: Drinking water is critical, some people even say to drink up to a gallon per day! It will flush your system of toxins and promote muscle growth. Your muscles are 70% water and some studies have indicated that even slight dehydration can lead to a 30% decrease in strength. So drink up. Add lemon to your water if you don't like just drinking plain water.

As an added bonus, drinking ice cold water has been shown to boost your metabolism because your body has to work harder to warm it and bring it to body temperature.

5). Avoid Stress: As discussed error, cortisol production is primarily stimulated by stress, so you want to avoid stress and sleep deprivation at all costs. Otherwise it will limit growth hormone and testosterone production and wreak all kinds of havoc on your body. It will also make your body less sensitive to insulin.

Luckily, you can counteract cortisol by learning to relax. Deep breathing techniques, getting proper sleep, reducing caffeine intake, getting quality nutrition, and cutting out alcohol can all help reduce stress.

6). Do Proper Exercises: It's been proven that short, intense workouts with short rest periods promote the production of growth hormone. That's why intense interval training is so great. Also, compound, multi-joint exercises like squats, lunges, pull-ups, deadlifts, bench presses, and overhead presses at high-intensity with minimal rest between sets increases the production of growth hormone and testosterone. Since the production of these hormones is proportional to intensity, you want to make sure that every workout you do is intense.

7). Take a Break from Working Out Every Few Months: It sounds strange, but lots of people report strength gains when they take a week or two off. That means no lifting weights or working out for an entire week. Some people get scared that they will lose their strength when they return to the gym, but that's just not the case.

In fact, this happened to me. I remember I got really sick one week and couldn't workout for over a week. I was really worried that I'd lose my strength and have to start up again using lower weights. Oddly enough, I noticed my arms looking bigger and more muscular... after not working out for over a week! When I started looking into it, I noticed that lots of people find that they have better strength gains when they take a break for at least 7 days. It's strange but true.

8). Fast Every Once in a While: If you eat too much, your insulin levels can rise, causing your body to stop producing human growth hormone. If you eat every few hours insulin levels can increase too much causing your body to stop producing human growth hormone. So insulin could be described as a fat storage hormone where human growth hormone could be described as a fat releasing hormone. So since insulin helps get glucose and nutrients into your muscles (or convert them into fat), when insulin levels are lower, human growth hormone levels will increase and turn stored fat into energy. Intermittent fasting is a great way to trigger this process. Fasting every once in a while, when you don't eat during the day will help you lose weight and still maintain muscle mass. .

The Actual Workouts

So by now we've covered quite a bit of information including the difference between training for strength and training for mass, the difference between compound full body workouts and split part workouts, the optimal amount of rest for strength or muscle gain, the 7 main exercises you'll do (plus their multiple variations), the progressive overload principle, and why complexes and circuits are great for losing weight and maintaining muscle.

So now I'm going to delve into actual workouts you can follow. These are all top notch programs that will help you with whatever goals you have. Whether you want to build muscle or shed fat, these will help you do just that. You'll notice that they all include weight lifting as well as cardio. That's because you really have to do both if you want to get ripped.

Here are a few important guidelines before you start:

1. **Start Light, Do It Right**: Before you start lifting heavy weights, start with a light weight and master the form. Doing an exercise will improper form will injure you, potentially preventing you from working out for weeks. Choose challenging weights that you can comfortably manage.
2. **Always Warm Up**: Foreplay happens before sex. Appetizers are before your meal. So why would it be any different for working out? Warming up will enhance coordination, flexibility, mobility, and help prevent injury. A good rule of thumb is to warm up for 5-10 minutes before your actual workout and to use about 15-25% of the actual weight you'll be lifting.
3. **Eat Quality Protein After Your Workout**: This can be a tuna salad, a piece of steak, or simply a whey protein shake.
4. **Follow the Workout**: If you want to see results, you have to choose a program and stick to it for at least 8 weeks. Of course you'll be adding weight, reducing rest intervals, varying the exercises so you don't plateau, but it's important to follow the program if you want to see results.

5. **Remember the 3 "Secrets" of the Fitness Industry**: Everything works. Nothing Works forever. Most workouts are the same. For the most part, most workouts are the same. The only thing that really changes are the weights, rest intervals, reps, and movement patterns. Unless you're an advanced level athlete or professional bodybuilder, most workout programs will produce plenty of results for you. .

Simple "Get Ripped" Workout

Here's a simple, no-nonsense workout that anyone can do in about 45 minutes (if not less). It only requires 5 basic exercises and is extremely functional and was created by strength coach Jason Ferrugia for "**Details**" magazine.

- Warm up using 15% to 25% of your actual work weight
- Workout three times a week, alternating between workout A and workout B
- Do cardio in between the weight lifting days
- Add 5 pounds of weight every week
- Follow this for 8 weeks

Note: Form is really important, so click on the links to see descriptions and video of the workouts

Workout A

Pull-ups: do as many as you can, stopping one repetition shy of failure for 4 sets. Rest 60 seconds between sets

Squats: Do 3 sets of 8 repetitions. Rest two minutes between sets

Overhead Press: Do 3 sets of 8 repetitions. Rest 60 seconds between sets

Workout B

Bench Press: Do 3 sets of 8 repetitions. Rest 60 seconds between sets

Farmers Walk: Grab two heavy dumbbells (45 to 75 pounds) and walk straight for 30 seconds, that's one set. Do 4 sets like this and rest for 90 seconds between sets

Deadlift: Do 4 sets of 4-8 repetitions. Rest two minutes between sets.

Cardio (on your non-weight lifting days)

Do 30 seconds of burpees, followed by 30 seconds of running in place, followed by 30 seconds of mountain climbers. Rest for 60 seconds and repeat 3 times.

Progress Chart: Week ____

Pull-ups: ____ Reps _____ Sets _____ Seconds rest between sets

Squats: Weight _____ lbs. _____ Reps ____ Sets ____ Seconds between sets

Overhead Press: Weight _____ lbs. ____ Reps ____ Sets ____ Seconds between sets

---

Bench Press: Weight _____ lbs. _____ Reps ____ Sets ____ Seconds between sets

Farmers Walk: Weight _____ lbs. ____ Reps ____ Sets ____ Seconds between sets

Deadlift: ____ Reps _____ Sets _____ Seconds rest between sets

---

Pull-ups: _____ Reps _____ Sets _____ Seconds rest between sets

Squats: Weight _____ lbs. _____ Reps _____ Sets _____ Seconds between sets

Overhead Press: Weight _____ lbs. _____ Reps _____ Sets _____ Seconds between sets

---

Bench Press: Weight _____ lbs. _____ Reps _____ Sets _____ Seconds between sets

Farmers Walk: Weight _____ lbs. _____ Reps _____ Sets _____ Seconds between sets

Deadlift: _____ Reps _____ Sets _____ Seconds rest between sets

Substitutions

Your body will adapt to the workout within 3 weeks, so you want to make slight modifications to the movements. If you recall, these movements are variations of the "Supreme 7" I mentioned in an earlier chapter. I'm linking to videos and descriptions of these exercises as well.

Here's how you'll modify these exercises:

Pull-ups: Modify the grip to a wide grip, facing palms toward you, or away from you

Squats: Barbell lunge or front squat

Overhead Press: Alternating shoulder press or dumbbell press

Deadlift: Snatch-grip deadlift or Romanian deadlift

Bench Press: Close grip bench press or incline bench press

Classic "5x5" Strength Workout

This workout is an absolute classic. It was popularized by Arnold Schwarzenegger before he became a bodybuilder. It is AMAZING for triggering myofibrillar hypertrophy (strength) without building bulky muscles. It's very similar to the previous workout, except that the rest is longer and the weight are much heavier. It's called "5x5" because it uses 5 sets of 5 reps per exercise.

- Do two warm up sets using 15% to 25% of your actual work weight
- Workout three times a week, alternating between workout A and workout B
- Do cardio in between the weight lifting days
- Add 5 lbs. per workout - but make sure you're lifting heavy (80% of your max)
- Follow this for 12 weeks, you WILL get strong - guaranteed

Note: Form is really important, so click on the links to see descriptions and video of the workouts

Workout A

Squats: Do 5 sets of 5 repetitions. Rest four to five minutes between sets

Bench Press: Do 5 sets of 5 repetitions. Rest four to five minutes between sets

Bentover Rows: Do 5 sets of 5 repetitions. Rest four to five minutes between sets

Workout B

Squats: Do 5 sets of 5 repetitions. Rest four to five minutes between sets

Overhead Press: Do 5 sets of 5 repetitions. Rest four to five minutes between sets

Deadlift: Do 1 set of 5 repetitions. Rest four to five minutes between sets

Cardio (on your non-weight lifting days)

Do 30 seconds of burpees, followed by 30 seconds of running in place, followed by 30 seconds of mountain climbers. Rest for 60 seconds and repeat 3 times.

Progress Chart: Week ____

Squats: Weight _____ lbs. _____ Reps
_____ Sets _____ Seconds between sets

Bench Press: Weight _____ lbs. _____ Reps
_____ Sets _____ Seconds between sets

Bentover Rows: Weight _____ lbs. _____ Reps _____ Sets ____ Seconds between sets

---

Squats: Weight _____ lbs. _____ Reps
_____ Sets _____ Seconds between sets

Overhead Press: Weight _____ lbs. _____ Reps _____ Sets _____ Seconds between sets

Deadlifts: Weight _____ lbs. _____ Reps
_____ Sets ____ Seconds between sets

Squats: Weight _____ lbs. _____ Reps _____ Sets _____ Seconds between sets

Bench Press: Weight _____ lbs. _____ Reps _____ Sets _____ Seconds between sets

Bentover Rows: Weight _____ lbs. _____ Reps _____ Sets _____ Seconds between sets

---

Squats: Weight _____ lbs. _____ Reps _____ Sets _____ Seconds between sets

Overhead Press: Weight _____ lbs. _____ Reps _____ Sets _____ Seconds between sets

Deadlifts: Weight _____ lbs. _____ Reps _____ Sets ____ Seconds between sets

---

Notes about the 5x5 Workout

This is a classic strength (myofibrillar hypertrophy) workout. Make no mistake, you will see great results.

It's critical to stick to the five reps and the 4-5 minutes of rest between sets. Because of the progressively heavy weight you'll be lifting, you are going to need to maintain proper form.

Going above 5 reps will compromise your form because of fatigue. Otherwise you run the risk of injury as you lift heavier weights.

Perform the movements quickly as this will help not only build strength but power as well.

Don't worry about the lack of "isolation" exercises because bench presses will build strong chest and triceps and rows will build really strong biceps.

Get rest between weight lifting days because this is a real strength workout which will tax your central nervous system (strength is a function of the CNS)

Home Dumbbell Workout

Here's another simple, no-nonsense workout that anyone can do in about 45 minutes (if not less). It's great for people that don't have access to a gym. All you need is a pair of dumbbells. I bought a 30lb pair for $30 from Craigslist. Then I got a pair of 40lb dumbbells as well.

- Warm up doing 10 bodyweight squats, 15 pushups, and 5 pull-ups (if you can)
- It uses variations of the "Supreme 7" movements to build muscle and burn fat
- This is an intense, calorie torching circuit
- Do 3 circuits in total

Dumbbell Stiff-Legged Deadlift: Do as many as you can for 30 seconds. Rest for 15 seconds then go to the next exercise.

Renegade Row: Do as many as you can for 30 seconds. Rest for 15 seconds then go to the next exercise.

Dumbbell Front Squat with Push Press:
Do as many as you can for 30 seconds. Rest for 15 seconds then go to the next exercise.

Sumo High Pull: Do as many as you can for 30 seconds. Rest for 15 seconds then go to the next exercise.

Mountain Climber: Do as many as you can for 30 seconds. Rest for 15 seconds then go to the next exercise.

Alternating Split Squats: Do as many as you can for 30 seconds. Rest for 15 seconds then go to the next exercise.

T-Pushups: Do as many as you can for 30 seconds. Rest for 15 seconds then go to the next exercise.

Repeat this circuit 3 times.

.

Progress Chart: Week ____

<u>Dumbbell Stiff-Legged Deadlift</u>: _____ Reps _____Sets _____ Seconds rest between sets

<u>Renegade Row</u>: Weight _____ lbs. _____ Reps _____ Sets _____ Seconds between sets

<u>Dumbbell Front Squat with Push Press</u>:
Weight _____ lbs. _____ Reps _____ Sets ____ Seconds between sets

<u>Sumo High Pull</u>: Weight _____ lbs. _____ Reps _____ Sets _____ Seconds between sets

<u>Mountain Climber</u>: Weight _____ lbs. _____ Reps _____ Sets ____ Seconds between sets

<u>Alternating Split Squats</u>: _____ Reps _____Sets _____ Seconds rest between sets

<u>T-Pushups</u>: Weight _____ lbs. _____ Reps _____ Sets _____ Seconds between sets

**Try to increase the number of sets you do (from 3 to 4) or increase the weight to further build muscle and strength..

Scientifically Simple Muscle Gain
This is an incredible workout created by world-renowned strength coach Joel Marion. It is a great blend of the principles you've learned thus far. And it's probably my favorite muscle building routine because of its' simplicity and efficiency. His clients (and his friends' clients) have seen tremendous gains in muscle mass and size.

The great thing about this workout is that it combines BOTH high rep (for muscle mass) and low rep (for greater strength) ranges to really get you great results - fast. Also, it's a full body workout, which is awesome for time-pressed people. If you follow this workout, you WILL see incredible results.

It focuses on 3 main principles:

1. Protect the central nervous system from getting burned out
2. Stimulate your muscles as much as safely possible (keeping point #1 in mind)
3. Doing a high volume to promote maximum muscle growth (hypertrophy)

It's a 40 minute workout that you do 5 times a week. This full body workout is comprised of the following movements:

Upper body horizontal push: Bench press (flat, incline, close-grip, or with dumbbells)

Upper body horizontal pull: Rows (bent over, one-arm dumbbell row, or seated row)

Upper body vertical push: Overhead press (standing press, push press, push jerk, dips, close-grip push press)

Upper body vertical pull: Pull-ups or lateral pulldowns

Quad-dominant lower body: Squats (back squat, front squat, or lunge) **Hip-dominant lower body** — Deadlift (sumo, conventional, Romanian, sumo squat) You'll alternate between the A movement of Group 1, then perform the B movement via straight sets. Repeat for Group 2. Here's how that would work:

Group 1
A1) Upper body horizontal push - 5 sets of 5 reps
A2) Upper body horizontal pull - 5 sets of 5 reps
B) Quad-dominant lower body - 5 sets of 5 reps

Group 2
A1) Upper body vertical push - 4 sets of 10 reps
A2) Upper body vertical pull - 4 sets of 10 reps
B) Hip-dominant lower body - 4 sets of 10 reps

Then you will switch the sets and reps (Group 1 does 4 sets of 10 reps and Group 2 does 5 sets of 5 reps) So here's an example of how that would look:

Monday
Group 1 5x5
Group 2 4x10

Tuesday
Group 1 4x10
Group 2 5x5

Thursday
Group 1 5x5
Group 2 4x10

Friday
Group 1 4x10
Group 2 5x5

You want to change the exercises every 3 weeks, so just choose a different variation of the exercise from each group so your body is constantly forced to grow and adapt. Marion recommends getting 5 workouts in per week. Try it out for 6 weeks and watch your muscles grow. After that do 3 sets of 5 reps and 5 sets of 8 reps.

.

Progress Chart: Week ____

Group 1
A1) Bench Press: Weight _____lbs. _____ Reps _____Sets _____ Seconds rest between sets

A2) Bentover row: Weight _____lbs. _____ Reps _____Sets _____ Seconds rest between sets

B) Back squat: Weight _____lbs. _____ Reps _____Sets _____ Seconds rest between sets

Group 2
A1) Dip: Weight _____lbs. _____ Reps _____Sets _____ Seconds rest between sets

A2) Pull-up: Weight _____lbs. _____ Reps _____Sets _____ Seconds rest between sets

B) Dumbbell swing: Weight _____lbs. _____ Reps _____Sets _____ Seconds rest between sets

For this workout, be sure to switch the sets and reps between 5x5 and 4x10 every workout..

Explosive Power Circuit Workout

So here's a workout I used to build power. You can see, that it uses Olympic movements of the snatch and jerk. You'll also notice that it's a full body workout that usually ends with an explosive bodyweight exercise like burpees or box jumps. This workout is GREAT for building explosive power.

- Warm up: some pushups, squats, and pull-ups will do the trick
- Choose challenging weights and increase by 5 lbs. each week
- Do all 3 exercises immediately after each other and take 1 minute rest; do this circuit 4 times
- Follow this for 3 weeks and then substitute the exercises

Monday

Squats: Do 8 repetitions and then go to the next exercise

Dumbbell Press: do 8 repetitions then go to the next exercise

Burpees: Do 8 repetitions and then rest for 60 seconds (more if you have to)

Wednesday

One Arm Dumbbell Power Snatch: Do 8 repetitions then go to the next exercise

One Arm Dumbbell Push Jerk: Do 8 repetitions then go to the next exercise

Box Jumps: Do 8 of these and then rest for 60 seconds (more if you have to)

Friday

Romanian Deadlifts: Do 8 and then go to the next exercise

Dumbbell High Pulls: Do 8 and then go to the next exercise

Lunges w/ Alternating Dumbbell Presses: Do 8 and then go to the next exercise

Dumbbell Hang Clean and Squat: Do 8 and then rest for 60 seconds

Cardio (on your non-weight lifting days)

Do 30 seconds of burpees, followed by 30 seconds of running in place, followed by 30 seconds of mountain climbers. Rest for 60 seconds and repeat 3 times.

Progress Chart: Week ____

Squats: _____ Reps _____ Sets

Dumbbell Press: Weight _____ lbs.
_____ Reps ____ Sets ____ Seconds between sets

Burpees: _____ Reps _____ Sets
_____ Seconds between sets

One Arm Power Snatch: Weight _____ lbs.
_____ Reps _____ Sets
_____ Seconds between sets

One Arm Push Jerk: Weight _____ lbs.
_____ Reps _____ Sets
_____ Seconds between sets

Box Jumps: _____ Reps _____ Sets _____ Seconds rest between sets

---

Romanian Deadlifts: _____ Reps _____ Sets _____ Seconds rest between sets

Dumbbell High Pull: Weight _____ lbs. _____ Reps _____ Sets _____ Seconds between sets

Lunges w/ Alternating Dumbbell Presses: Weight _____ lbs. _____ Reps _____ Sets ___ Seconds between sets

Dumbbell Hang Clean and Squats: Weight _____ lbs. _____ Reps _____ Sets _____ Seconds rest between sets

Substitutions

Your body will adapt to the workout within 3 weeks, so you want to make slight modifications to the movements. If you recall, these movements are variations of the "Supreme 7" I mentioned in an earlier chapter. I'm linking to videos and descriptions of these exercises as well.

Here's how you'll modify these exercises:

Squats: Barbell lunge or front squat

Box Jumps: Jump squats

Dumbbell Press: Overhead press (with barbell).

Explosive Power Circuit Workout

Here's a GREAT periodized strength training workout. It will help get you bigger and stronger and was developed by world renowned strength coach and author Elliott Hulse. He uses it for the football players at his "Strength Camp". It will help you build strength, size, and power.

- Warm up: some pushups, squats, and pull-ups will do the trick
- Choose challenging weights and increase by 5 lbs. each week
- Do all 3 exercises immediately after each other and take 1 minute rest; do this circuit 4 times
- Follow this for 3 weeks and then substitute the exercises

Monday

Bench Press: Do 6 sets of 3 repetitions (heavier weight)

Bodybuilding Circuit: Do 8 dumbell incline bench presses, followed immediately by 8 seated rows, followed immediately by 8 upright rows then rest for 2 minutes and repeat this 3 times

Ab Rollouts: Do 8 repetitions and then rest for 60 seconds (more if you have to)

Wednesday
Front Squats : Do 6 sets of 3 repetitions (heavier weight)

Bodybuilding Circuit: Do 6 repetitions of straight-leg deadlift, followed immediately by 6 repetitions of dumbbell stepups, followed immediately by reverse woodchops, followed immediately by 6 repetitions of renegade rows then rest for 2 minutes and repeat 3 times

Bar Hold: Hold 225 pounds for as long as you can (this will build great grip strength)

Friday
Power Cleans: Do 5 sets of 5 repetitions

Farmer Walk: Do 5 repetitions of these

Dumbbell Pushups: Do 3 sets of as many reps as possible

Inverted Rows: Do 3 sets of as many reps as possible.

Cardio (on your non-weight lifting days)
Do 30 seconds of burpees, followed by 30 seconds of running in place, followed by 30 seconds of mountain climbers. Rest for 60 seconds and repeat 3 times.

·

Progress Chart: Week ____

Bench Press: _____ Reps _____ Sets

Bodybuilding Circuit: Weight _____ lbs. _____ Reps _____ Sets
_____ Seconds between sets

Ab Rollouts: _____ Reps _____ Sets
_____ Seconds between sets

Front Squats: Weight _____ lbs. _____ Reps _____ Sets _____ Seconds between sets

Bodybuilding Circuit: Weight _____ lbs. _____ Reps _____ Sets
_____ Seconds between sets

Bar Hold: _____ Reps _____ Sets _____ Seconds rest between sets

---

Power Cleans: _____ Reps _____ Sets
_____ Seconds rest between sets

Farmer Walk: Weight _____ lbs. _____ Reps _____ Sets _____ Seconds between sets

Dumbbell Pushups: Weight _____ lbs. _____ Reps _____ Sets _____ Seconds between sets

Inverted Rows: Weight _____ lbs. _____ Reps _____ Sets _____ Seconds rest between sets

18 Mindblowing Nutrition Tips for Busy Guys to Get Ripped

Nutrition is one of the most controversial subjects in the fitness industry. There are so many contradictory opinions out there, the average guy can't keep up.

There's the Atkins diet, Paleo diet, South Beach Diet, and literally dozens of others. Often times, there are big controversies in the diet/nutrition industry:

- Breakfast vs no breakfast for fatloss
- Working out fed vs fasted
- Low carb vs high carb dilemma
- Multiple meals vs intermittent fasting

Plus, I'm not a big fan on giving out diets and eating plans because they're so hard to keep up with. I mean, if you're a guy like me, you have family gatherings, barbeques with friends and neighbors, business lunches, and kid's birthday parties on nearly a weekly basis. How are you supposed to stick to a pre-calculated meal plan with such a busy life? It's just not practical. Plus, there's so much evidence showing that people who stick to diets slide back into their old eating habits and gain their weight back.

I read on the ScrawnytoBrawny.com blog:

> *"Give me a one-page bullet-list of exactly what I should do. That's worth more to me than a stack of books that I have to dig through to get to the good stuff. I may give you 50 bucks for the books. But I'll pay you $5,000 for the one page."*

That's a quote from Alwyn Cosgrove, a world-famous strength coach and entrepreneur.

So I'm giving you this cheat sheet of some of my favorite nutrition hacks and tips. They focus on lifestyle changes and principles that you can fit into your busy life.

1.). **Eliminate All Drinks Except Water**: Gatorade, sports drinks, cola's, alcohol, etc. add unneccesary calories to your diet. You should be drinking at least 2 liters of water per day. This will help you lose weight and detoxify your body, flush out your kidneys, etc. Adding lemon to your water is a great way to add flavor and further aid in detoxifying your body.

I just buy a 1 liter re-usable bottle of water and drink one full bottle in the morning before lunch and one bottle after lunch. I'll then drink one or two cups of green tea or coffee and that's nearly 3 liters of water right there.

One more thing, even though water will seem bland compared to the other drinks you may be used to drinking, after drinking water for about a week you won't really want that sugary stuff. Plus, if you add lemon to your water, your tastebuds will be more sensitive to the flavor, so it'll taste better.

2). **Eliminate Sugar and Starchy Carbs From Your Diet**: This is a big one too. Simply removing donuts, cup cakes, chips, cookies, candy bars, jelly beans, etc. will have a tremendous impact in helping you get in shape. You'll likely drop a few pounds in a few weeks just by making these tweaks. Sugary, processed carbs are really high in calories and very low in nutritional value, plus they don't satisfy your hunger... unless you eat a lot. So stay away from all of those boxed snacks and junk food products... even the "low fat" versions because they usually add sugar or high-fructose corn syrup to make them taste better.

I know this sounds like common sense, but just eat one ingredient foods (almonds, berries, eggs, meat, fish, green peppers, etc.)

3). **Eat Lots of Vegetables**: Many people don't eat enough vegetables. Vegetables have lots of fiber which is great for your digestive system, lowering cholesterol, etc. Also, they have anti-oxidants that help fight cancer. As an added benefit, they keep you fuller longer and help you feel more satisfied after a meal.

I like to sautee vegetables in garlic and a little bit of salt. That's a GREAT way to make them taste really good.

4). **Eat Enough Protein**: High-protein diets not only promote muscle hypertrophy (growth) but they also enhance fat loss. Researchers at Skidmore College (Saratoga Springs, New York) found that subjects following a high- protein diet–40% of total daily calories from protein–for 8 weeks lost significantly more body fat, especially abdominal fat, than those following a low-fat/high-carb diet. One explanation for these findings is that more protein boosts levels of peptide YY, a hormone that is produced by gut cells that travel to the brain to decrease hunger and increase satiety.

5). **Avoid Refined Carbs**: Carbs are NOT the enemy. You just have to eat the right kinds at the right time. When you eat carbs, choose slow-digesting whole grains such as brown rice, oatmeal and whole-wheat bread, which keep insulin levels low and steady, and help prevent insulin spikes from stopping the fat-burning process and ramping up fat-storing. .

A study conducted by scientists at Pennsylvania State University found that participants following a low-calorie diet with carbs coming from whole grains lost significantly more abdominal fat than people following a low-calorie diet with refined carbs.

6). **Fat is Important**: Fat gets a bad wrap. Some fats, like omega-3's can help promote fat loss. Eating fats to lose fat might seem counterintuitive, but choosing "good" fat sources like salmon, sardines, trout, olive oil, peanut butter, walnuts, etc. can actually help you burn fat compared to if you went on a low fat diet. One of the reasons fat is so important is because it helps tell your body that you're full. If you strip fat from your diet, you'll sabotage your weight loss goals because you'll always feel unsatisfied.

7). **Eat Whole Eggs**: Eggs provide high amounts of protein and cholesterol. Profein helps you build muscle and stay fuller longer and cholesterol is a key building block of testosterone, so it's also key for building muscle. Not only are eggs packed with protein, they have been shown to promote muscle strength and mass. Furthermore, research shows that people consuming eggs for breakfast helped subjects eat fewer calories throughout the rest of the day and also lose significantly more body fat. So go ahead and hard boil some eggs and keep them on hand, or have scrambled eggs with lots of vegetables and some hot sauce.

8). **Eat More Grapefruit**: Research from the Scripps Clinic (San Diego) showed that subjects who ate half a grapefruit or drank 8 ounces of grapefruit juice three times a day while eating normally lost approximately 4 pounds in 12 weeks. Some subjects lost up to 10 pounds without dieting. This is likely due to grapefruit's ability to lower insulin levels. You can simply add half a grapefruit to some of your meals.

9). **Use Spicy Condiments**: Cholula, Lousiana hot sauce, crushed red peppers, chili ginger paste, etc. not only adds tons of flavor to your meals, it helps promote better calorie burning. The effects are even enhanced when you consume caffeine.

10). **Eat Avocadoes**: Avocados have lots of monounsaturated fat, which isn't typically stored as body fat. They also contain a compound called mannoheptulose, that actually blunts insulin release and helps enhance calcium

absorption. Keeping insulin low is critical for encouraging fat loss, and adequate calcium can promote fat loss as well.

11). **Drink Green Tea**: Having one or two cups of green tea per day is a good idea. The main ingredient found in green tea, epigallocatechin gallate (EGCG), helps inhibit the enzyme that breaks down the neurohormone norepinephrine. Norepinephrine helps keep the metabolic rate up, so by drinking green tea, you burn more calories throughout the day. Drinking green tea is also a great way to stay hydrated during your workouts. A study in The Journal of Nutrition reported that subjects who drank green tea and consistently exercised lost significantly more abdominal fat than subjects who drank a placebo.

12). **Drink Ice Water**: German researchers have discovered that drinking about 2 cups of ice cold water temporarily boosts metabolic rate by roughly 30%. The reason appears to be mainly because of an increase in norepinephrine. In fact, Tim Ferriss, in his 4 Hour Body book talks about talking cold ice baths to boost your metabolism as well. The theory is that your body is forced to warm itself up, which burns calories.

13). **Avoid Artificial Sweeteners**: Although artificially sweetened drinks are calorie-free, drinking too much of that stuff can actually hurt your fat-loss progress. Beverages like diet soda mess with your brain's ability to regulate calorie intake, causing you to feel hungrier than normal so you eat more total calories.

14). **Be Smart About Portions**: A study from Cornell University reported that moviegoers who were given a large container (about 22 cups) of popcorn during a movie, ate 45% more than moviegoers given a medium container. Even subjects given a large container of stale popcorn still ate about 35% more than those given a medium container, even though they thought the popcorn tasted bad. A smart way to interpret this research is for lean protein sources, serve yourself a large amount; for side dishes like rice, potatoes and bread, keep the servings on the small side.

In general, you want your diet to consist of 40% carbs, 30% protein, and 30% fat. Now this will vary a little based, but these are pretty solid numbers. If you eat the right foods, hitting these macronutrient targets won't be hard… and you won't feel hungry.

15). **Use an App**: It's hard to calculate your daily macronutrients for the busy guy. That's why it's a great idea to use an app like FitDay.com or MyFitnessPal.com to give you a good idea of how much you're eating.

For the most part, eating the right, healthy foods will automatically get your macronutrients in line.

16). **More Carbs on Lifting Days**: Like I mentioned in the main manual, you want to eat more carbs on your weight lifting days, preferably AFTER lifting weights to replenish your glycogen stores. Stick with good carbs like sweet potatoes, russet potatoes, jasmine rice, etc.

17). **Combine Protein and Carbs**: A smart way of eating is to pair protein with carbs. So eating potatoes and protein will help lessen the insulin spike that the carbs would trigger if eaten alone. Plus, adding some vegetables like broccoli, green beans, kale, spinach, peppers, etc. will round off that meal. .

18).**You Don't Have to Be Perfect**: Professional models diet down, get airbrushed, get all kinds of implants (I'm talking about men; calf implants, pec implants, bicep implants, etc.) so don't feel like you have to follow a meal plan perfectly. For the most part, if you eat right 85% to 95% of the time, you'll see great results.

Five Great Protein Sources

- Eggs
- Chicken breast
- Lean steak
- Extra-lean ground turkey
- Greek yogurt

Seven Great Vegetables

- Broccoli
- Spinach
- Green beans
- Carrots
- Zucchini
- Green Peppers
- Kale

Five Great Complex Carbohydrate Sources

- Brown rice
- Quinoa
- Sweet potatoes
- Yams
- Steel cut oatmeal

Five Great Fat Sources

- Raw nuts
- All natural nut buttervocado
- Olive oil
- Homemade salad dressing

Common Form Mistakes

Please read this very carefully, especially if you haven't lifted weights before, or if it's been a long time. The motto "keep it light until you get it right" might sound cheesy, but it's extremely important.

The biggest thing that will kill your progress is an injury. I've hurt my knee, shoulder, and hip before by not lifting correctly. As you increase your weights, you have to be hyper-focused on form. Thankfully, my injuries healed within a few days, so they didn't stop me from working out, but they were a very good reminder of how important proper form is. I have friends who have hurt their back and shoulders and now can't do any weight lifting. I don't want this to happen to you, so please read this short guide carefully and check out the links I've included.

I could have taken pictures and videos of myself doing the exercises, but there are a bunch of REALLY great resources online for that already. They helped me immensely, so I'm sharing them with you as well.

Bench Press

Make Sure You Do the Following:

- Squeeze the bar really hard
- Keep your elbows in, close to your body to prevent shoulder injuries
- Grip the bar slightly wider than shoulder width apart
- Lift across your nipple line; the bar should touch your chest at the nipple
- Keep your back arched; someone should be able to slide their arm under your lower back
- Squeeze your shoulder blades together
- Keep your feet spread apart
- Inhale as you lower the weight, exhale as you lift it back up

DON'T Do the Following:

- Don't lift more weight than you can handle
- Don't worry about what other guys in the gym will think about you
- Don't spread your arms out too wide; shoulder width apart is best for beginners
- Don't bounce the bar off your chest; lower it in a controlled fashion, but then explosively lift it back up

Here's an [excellent bench press tutorial](#) here's [another good one](#).

Overhead Press

The overhead press is a great exercise that you don't see a lot of guys doing in the gym. Doing it properly will provide immense strength and muscle building benefits.

Make Sure You Do the Following:

- Start with your feet shoulder width apart
- Grab the bar slightly wider than your shoulders
- Grip the bar very tight
- Keep your chest up
- Move your head back slighly as you lift the bar, then push your head back forward again
- Lift the weight straight up and lock your arms
- Keep your entire body (core, back, and legs) tight

DON'T Do the Following:

- Don't lift more weight than you can handle Overhead pressing is actually a pretty safe exercise. It's great for your shoulders (compared to the bench press). Here's a great article with pictures and a video.

    http://doubleyourgains.com/how-to-overhead-press

    http://bit.ly/1WEZEhm.

Squat

Squats are one of the best exercises you can do for your body. Since your quadriceps, hamstrings, and glutes are the biggest muscles in your body, working these will trigger a strong release of growth hormone in your body, allowing you to gain muscle and burn fat.

I've personally hurt myself squatting incorrectly, so please follow these instructions very carefully

Make Sure You Do the Following:

- Use a weight that you can handle
- Put the bar on your traps (you'll have to squeeze your shoulder blades together and flare out your lats)
- Squeeze the bar as hard as you can
- As you hold the bar, your elbows should be pointing down (not back)
- Inhale and fill your abdomen (don't inhale and inflate your chest)
- Keep your back as upright as possible
- Lower the weight by moving your butt out
- As you go down, be sure to push your knees out (don't let them buckle in)
- Make sure your thighs are parallel to the ground before you come back up

- Try to keep your back straight
- When you push up, push down through your heels (NOT from your toes)

DON'T Do the Following:

- Under no circumstances should you let your knees buckle in; if this happens then make a conscious effort to push them out as you squat down
- Don't lean forward too much; if you are then you probably are squatting too much weight
- Don't hold your breath; be sure to exhale as you come back up
- Don't do half squats or quarter squats; doing full squats is better for your knees because you develop your muscles equally and in a balanced manner

Here is a good squat tutorial

http://www.bodybuilding.com/exercises/detail/view/name/barbell-full-squat

This is the best squat tutorial I've ever read. It's brief and once I did what he said, I was able to squat without injuring myself. .

http://jasonferruggia.com/how-to-squat-properly/

Deadlift

Deadlifts are an amazing exercise because they work all of the muscles in your body with the heaviest weight possible. But it's a double-edged sword because you can hurt yourself if you don't do them right.

Make Sure You Do the Following:

- The bar should be above your feet on the floor
- Grip the bar as hard as you can
- Your stance should be shoulder width apart
- Bend your knees so your shins touch the bar
- KEEP YOUR BACK STRAIGHT
- Lift through your knees and pull up
- A point that many people don't know is to flex your glutes hard toward the end of the movement. This is really important for stabilizing your entire body.

Here's an excellent tutorial and video of the deadlift. Notice how he keeps his back perfectly straight and how his knees and hips extend at the same time. It just looks so crisp.

http://stronglifts.com/how-to-deadlift-with-proper-technique/

http://bit.ly/1mGY63f

Free Bonus Report

Can I Ask You a Quick Favor (again)?

If you like this book, I would **greatly appreciate** if you could leave an honest review on Amazon.

Reviews are very important to us authors, and it only takes a minute to post.

Also, don't forget to check out my new book:

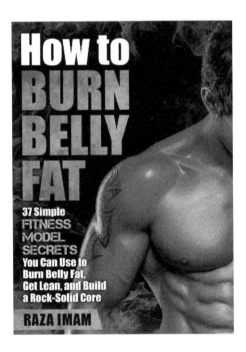

Printed in Great Britain
by Amazon